Lessons in Practising Yoga

Lessons in Practising Yoga

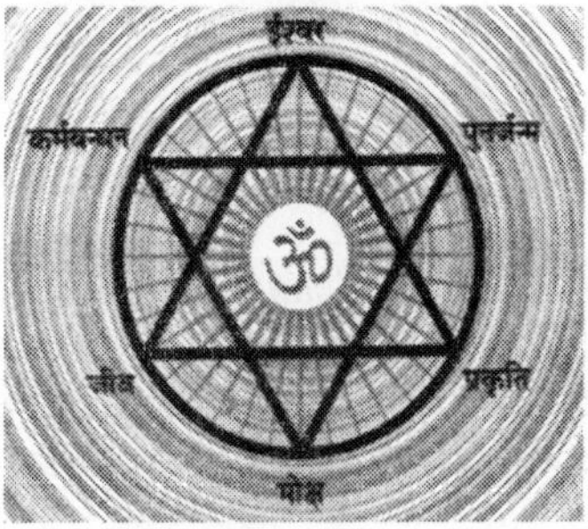

Vidya Sagar Verma
(Former Ambassador of India to Kazakhstan)

PRABHAT PAPERBACKS

संकल्प
An organisation dedicated to inculcate social commitment amongst Civil Services aspirants

Published by
PRABHAT PAPERBACKS
4/19 Asaf Ali Road,
New Delhi-110 002 (INDIA)
e-mail: prabhatbooks@gmail.com

ISBN 978-93-5266-967-7
LESSONS IN PRACTISING YOGA
by Vidya Sagar Verma

Edition
First, 2018

Price
₹ 300.00 (Rupees Three Hundred only)

Printed at
R-Tech Offset Printers, Delhi

Dedicated
to
All Aspirants of Yoga

Dedication

I bow to God for inspiring in me
Sankalp to write 'Lessons in Practising Yoga'.
I bow to my Teachers who imbued in me
Love for Indian Culture and Philosophy.
Believing all have Divine Spark in them
With incessant craving for reaching the Divine,
Hoping the readers to rise above material pursuits
To follow the enlightening Yogic path sublime,
I dedicate this book to All Aspirants of Yoga
Praying for them Peace, Prosperity and Bliss Divine.

Prayer

(Inter – Faith Prayer For The Right Path)

TAT SAVITUR VAREÑYAM
BHARGO DEVASYA DHÎMAHI
DHIYO YO NAH PRACHODYÃT (1)

(Father of all!, may Thy supernal Light
Inspire, illuminate, and guide our minds!
We open them to let Thy Glory in.)
—Rig Veda 3.62.10

AGNE NAYA SUPATHÃ RÃYE ASMÃN
VISHVÃNI DEVA VAYUNÃNI VIDVÃN
YUYODHYASMAJ JUHURÃÑ MENO
BHÛYAŠTHÃN TE NAMAH UKTIM VIDHEMA (2)

(Supreme Director! Lord of Warmth and Light,
Of Life and Consciousness, that knowest all!
Guide us by the Right Path to happiness,
And give us strength and will to war against
The sins that rage in us and lead astray!
We bow in adoration unto Thee!)
—Yajur Veda 40.16

Grant us long life, Great Lord! And fortitude
And the right mind, and show us the Straight Path,
Over which Thou broodest, and which leads to Thee!
—Gatha (Zoroastrian Scripture)

Hear, O Lord!, my cry, give ear unto my prayer,
that goeth not out of feigned lips.
Hold up my goings in Thy Paths,
that my footsteps slip not.
Show me Thy Ways, O Lord! teach me Thy Paths;
and lead me in Thy Truth.
Thou art the God of my salvation.
Open Thou mine eyes that I may behold
wondrous things out of Thy Law.
Quicken Thou me according to Thy word.
Remove from me the way of lying.

—The Holy Bible

Lord of Compassion! All praise unto Thee!
Creator and Protector of the worlds!
Lord God! Beneficent and Merciful!
Master Supreme of the great Judgement Day!
Thee do we serve and Thee beseech for help;
Show us the Path on which Thy blessings rest;
The Straight Path; not of those who go astray,
On whom descend Thy wrath and punishment

—The Holy Quran

AUM ! AMEN ! AMIN! *

---

*'Aum' is a word sacred not only to the Hindus but also to the Buddhists, the Jains and the Sikhs. It is generally believed that it also has close etymological and spiritual links with the 'Amen' and 'Amin' of Christianity and Islam.

—Dr. Karan Singh

Rose is the symbol of Love. Marigold is the symbol of Devotion

Lotus is the symbol of Enlightenment. Lotus is the seat of Goddess Saraswati.

Accordingly, at the end of each Topic, Lotus flower has been printed.

—Author

In Praise of God

YASYEME HIMAVANTO MAHITVÃ
YASYA SAMUDRAM RASAYÃ SAHÃHUH
YASYEMAH PRADISHO YASYA BÃHÛ
KASMAI DEVÃYA HAVIŠÃ VIDHEMA (3)

(Whose glory the ice capped mountains sing
whose glory the oceans with rivers sing
whose arms, the directions, encompass the whole
that Lord of Creation, in obeisance we adore.)
(Rig Veda 10.121.4)

The heavens declare the glory of God
And the firmament showeth His handiwork
(The Holy Bible – Psalms 19.1)

Have you not seen that are in the skies —
The Sun, the Moon, the Stars, — and the Mountains
And animals and many men are in obeisance to Him ?
(The Holy Quran 22.18)

The Divine Promise

YUJE VÃM BRAHMA PÛRVYAM NAMOBHIRVI
SHLOKA ETU PATHYEVA SÛREH
SHRIÑVANTU VISHVE AMRITASYA PUTRÃH
Ã YE DHÃMÃNI DIVYÃNI TASTHUH (4)

(Listen! World's children of the Immortal
By Yoga you can attain heavenly abode.
Approach the enlightened and meditate on Me
I will lead you both to the Blissful state).
—Yajur Veda (11.5)

Knock, And It shall be opened unto you.
—The Holy Bible (Mathew: 7.7)

And I will give unto thee,
The keys of the Kingdom of Heaven
—The Holy Bible (Mathew: 16.19)

I am in your Souls! Why see ye not?
In every Breath of Yours am I, but ye
Are blind without true eye, and see me not
—The Holy Quran

—(The Essential Unity of All Religions Page 130):
Bhagwan Das

Message

I am deeply pleased that Sh. Vidya Sagar Verma, IFS Retd. has written a book 'Lessons in Practising Yoga'. I have had the pleasure of reading his earlier book 'Yoga Darshana : Kavya Vyakhya' (A poetical commentary in Hindi on the Yoga Sutras of Maharishi Patanjali).

I have known Ambassador Vidya Sagar Verma since 2010 when he joined us as senior faculty for the Interview Guidance Program for the aspirants of the Civil Services. Vidya Sagar ji is well versed in the Vedas, the Upanishads, the Gita and the Darshanas and has been promoting Indian Culture and Philosophy abroad with zeal and dedication. While Ambassador of India in Kazakhstan, he conducted Yoga classes in the Embassy premises which were attended by Kazakh nationals as also by some Kazakhstan based diplomats and their spouses. He also got translated the Bhagvad Gita, 1100 Mantras of Rig Veda and abridged Mahabharata into Kazakh language. For his dedicated service to Samkalp as also for his contribution in promoting Indian Culture and Philosophy, he was conferred 'Guru Samman' by Samkalp in July 2015.

Ambassador Verma's lectures in Yoga in Kazakhstan were compiled in a bilingual book 'Lessons in Practising Yoga' (English and Russian). On the suggestion of Samkalp, he has revised the English version of his book, keeping in mind the English knowing younger generation whose interest in Yoga has been aroused with the UN declaration of 21st June as International Day of Yoga.

The book imparts lessons not only in Yoga-Asanas and Pranayama but also in Moral Discipline and Meditation which is, in fact, the core of Yoga philosophy. In the days of blind pursuit of materialism, a dose of spirituality is extremely essential for introducing these deeper concepts to the younger generation.

I do hope that this book will help the aspirants of Yoga realise our daily prayer, which is the quintessence of all prayers: ASTO MÃ SAD GAMAYA ,TAMSO MÃ JYOTIR GAMAYA, MRITYOR MÃ AMRITAM GAMAYA (5), i.e. O God! Lead us from untruth to truth, from darkness to light and from mortality to immortality!

Santosh Kumar Taneja
Founder Samkalp

New Delhi
June 25, 2018

Thus Spake Swami Vivekananda

Today, as always, man seeks God – and often without knowing he is doing so. All human activity – good, bad, or indifferent – is actually the misapplied search for God.

The fact is that man in his true nature is already divine; but this divinity is covered. Life's one purpose is realisation of divinity.

Realisation of divinity is religion. At base, all religions teach this same truth although accretions often obscure it. Vedanta emphasises the one objective of realisation but accepts diverse methods of reaching it.

Realisation may be gained by the practice of the Yoga of knowledge, or of control of mind, or of selfless work, or of love of God – or by a combination of Yogas.

—(What Religion Is – In the Words of Swami Vivekananda)

Foreword

During the British rule, the services of renowned German Philosopher, Prof. F. Max Muller, who had not only studied Sanskrit language, the Vedas and the Upanishads, but also translated the Vedas and the Upanishads, were requisitioned to give lectures to the ICS officers selected to serve in India. The excellent and well-meaning lectures which he delivered to them, have been compiled in a book, India: What Can It Teach Us? On the basis of these studies, he commented in the very first lecture to the ICS officers:

"If I were to look over the whole world to find out the country most richly endowed with all the wealth, power and beauty that Nature can bestow – in some parts a very paradise on earth – I should point to India.

"If I were asked under what sky the human mind has most fully developed some of its choicest gifts, has most deeply pondered on the greatest problems of life, and has found solutions of some of them which well deserve the attention even of those who have studied Plato and Kant – I should point to India."

"And if I were to ask myself from what literature we, here in Europe, who have been nurtured almost exclusively on the thoughts of Greeks and Romans, and of one Semitic race, the Jewish, may draw that corrective which is most wanted in order to make our inner life more perfect, more comprehensive, more universal, in fact more truly human, a life, not for this life only, but a transfigured and eternal life – again I would point to India."

—India: What Can It Teach Us? (page 4)

Prof. Max Muller brought out the importance of studying and learning the Indian Culture and Civilisation as an aid to civil servants to administer the growth of the country

Samkalp is a social organisation whose avowed mission is to inculcate Integrity, Compassion, and Excellence among the aspiring civil servants. It not only imparts them lessons for preparing for the Civil Services for discharging their social responsibilities towards the people of the country as proud members of the Civil Services Examinations, it also conducts Interview Guidance Programmes by senior retired civil servants and others for the aspirants to clear the interview, as well as hold special lectures and personality development camps.

Another book worth reading is 'Lessons in Practising Yoga' authored by Sh. Vidya Sagar Verma, the retired Indian Foreign Service Officer who while serving as Ambassador in Kazakhstan conducted Yoga classes there which were attended by not only Kazakh nationals but also some foreign diplomats and their spouses resident in Kazakhstan. Sh. Vidya Sagar Verma has also authored a book 'Yoga Darshana – Kavya Vyakhya" (A Poetical Commentary in Hindi on all the Yoga Sutras of Sage Patanjali) which was released by the Hon. Vice President of India Sh. Krishna Kant in April 2002.

Due to the efforts of the Indian Government, UN declared in December 2014, 21st June as International Day of Yoga which is being celebrated enthusiastically all over the world since then. Now the young generation in our country has also got enthused to practise Yoga. But Yoga is not mere Yoga-Asanas and Breathing Exercises, it is much more, particularly its moral content. In the 195 Sutra Yoga treatise, there are only three sutras related to Asanas and six sutras related to Pranayama. All the rest relate to Moral Discipline and Meditation. This aspect of Yoga discipline has been duly emphasised by Rev. Albert Mohler Jr., thus: "You may be twisting yourself into pretzels or grass hoppers but if there is no meditation or direction of consciousness, you are not practising Yoga." Sh. Vidya Sagar has discussed comprehensively all aspects of Yoga philosophy in 'Lessons in Practising Yoga' in a simple way easily understood by everybody.

We hope that this book will help bring a great change in the lives of practitioners of Yoga. Yoga will develop in them physical, mental and moral faculties and bring immense peace and richness in their lives. Additionally, the civil servants who practise Yoga in all its aspects will be able to realise the Gita's dictum "**yogah karmsu kaushalam** " i.e perfection in action is yoga

Radhey Shyam Gupta, IPS (Retd.)
President, Samkalp

New Delhi
June 4, 2018

Preface

It gives me immense pleasure to present 'Lessons in Practising Yoga' for the English knowing young generation of India whose interest has been aroused by the declaration of 21st June as the International Day of Yoga by the United Nations. This book, in fact, is an enlarged edition of my bilingual (English – Russian) book of the same title which was published in Kazakhstan during my tenure (May 2002 to December 2004) there.

I have been practising Yoga and reading about its philosophy for the last five decades. During my assignment as High Commissioner of India to Papua New Guinea, I authored a book "Yoga Darshana Kavya Vyakhya' (a Poetical Commentary in Hindi on the Yoga Aphorisms of Sage Patanjali). This was brought out under the Golden Jubilee of India's Independence Series of the Rashtriya Sanskrit Sanasthan (Deemed University), New Delhi and released by the Hon. Vice President of India, Sh. Krishna Kant in April 2002.

My assignment as Ambassador of India to Kazakhstan had been very rewarding not only professionally, but also from the point of view of my love for Yoga. It is well known that the erstwhile Soviet Union had made in depth researches in Yoga and the psychic powers of the mind. I had read about this in the books like 'Psychic Discoveries Behind the Iron Curtain' by Sheila Ostrander and Lynn Schroeder and the 'The Search for Psychic Power' by David Hammond. The books are replete with detailed accounts of psychic researches by scientists of Kazakhstan, Ukraine and Russia.

It was, therefore, not surprising for me to meet in Kazakhstan a good number of people who expressed interest in learning Yoga, nor was it difficult to find Russian knowing Yoga teachers who received training in Yoga in Russia or Ukraine. Books on Yoga in Russian language were also available for their use.

Yoga classes were introduced free of charge in the Indian Cultural Centre of the Embassy. The course devised was of three months duration and each student was to atter.d two classes a week. Four classes of one hour duration each were conducted in the Embassy daily. The lessons in Yoga were imparted in all its aspects-Moral Discipline Physical Exercises, Breathing Exercises and Meditation. Over 1500 persons attended Yoga classes during my tenure in Kazakhstan.

To cater to the desire of some of my colleagues from the diplomatic community to learn Yoga, classes were started on every Saturday for them. The lessons in practising Yoga were imparted by me in English with simultaneous interpretation in Russian. A good number of diplomats, including some Heads of Missions and their spouses attended the classes.

Conduct of these classes also resulted in compilation of my lessons in a bilingual book 'Lessons in Practising Yoga' (English – Russian). The other pleasant by-product of this venture was that the Hindi version of these lessons along with detailed Sanskrit references on the relevant subject, was annexed as a separate section to the second edition of my book 'Yoga Darshana: Kavya Vyakhya', the utility of which has been further enhanced as it provides practical steps for practising Yoga.

The present book has been enlarged to include detailed Introduction to the Philosophy of Yoga as also detailed Introduction to the Ancient Indian Philosophy on which Yoga discipline is based. Apart from many relevant Sanskrit references, quotations of renowned philosophers as also from scriptures of the world's main religions have been included by way of comparative study. Sanskrit texts have been transliterated in Roman Script followed by translation in English. Those who find difficulty in reading Sanskrit text in Roman Script may skip it, if they so wish and proceed to the translation. The original Sanskrit texts in Devanagri Script have been given in the Annexure to the book, as per serial numbers indicated against each. **The purpose of quoting original texts is three-fold: first, it adds authenticity to what is being said; second, it provides glimpses of original texts to those who have not studied Sanskrit and three, it keeps the author on track, warding him off deviations and pouring in his own fanciful ideas on the subject.** In other words, what has been said in this book, is not mine – IDAM NA MAMA. All belongs to the renowned saints and sages of Yore.

I would like to heartily thank the worthy Founder of Samkalp. Shri Santosh Kumar Taneja and the President of Samkalp, Shri Radhey Shyam Gupta, IPS (Retd.) as also Samkalp's sister organization Jan-Kalyan Shiksha Samiti for bringing out this book under their ageis. Samkalp is a social organisation which imparts lessons/training to aspirants for civil services examination particularly to those who can ill afford to receive coaching in the concerned coaching institutes and academies. The motto of Samkalp is to enthuse Integrity, Compassion and Excellence among the aspirants of civil services who will be the engine for implementation of Government policies. I earnestly appreciate Samkalp's decision for gifting this book to the entrants to the civil services with a view to inculcating in them high moral values and helping them perform their duties as true servants of the people of India, adding lustre to the nomenclature 'Public Servant'.

I sincerely thank Shri Prabhat Kumar, Proprietor Prabhat Publications, New Delhi for preparing excellent design and layout and for publication of the book. I am deeply grateful to Shri Bihari Lal Singhal, Proprietor BB Press, Noida for his generous support in printing this book.

I have also used views of some modern Indian and Foreign scholars as also their diagrams and photographs on the subject, the sources of which I am not aware. I thank them all sincerely and profusely. I also thank Mr. Ruslan Rachmatulin, a Yoga Teacher in our Embassy in Kazakhstan for his photographs of Yoga Asanas appearing in the book. A few photographs are of my son Shashank.

I also thank Sh. Vijay Bhatia, former Manager, Punjab National Bank and Kumari Deepali of Samkalp for assisting in typing work. My daughter Archana and my grand daughter Ritambhara also helped in typing the Manuscript. I give them both and son Shashank my heart-felt Shubhãšĩsh to pursue the Yogic path in their lives.

I earnestly hope that this book will bring a great change in the lives of readers and practitioners of Yoga. Any small efforts made in this direction will never go waste and bring immense peace, satisfaction and fulfilment in their lives.

Gautam Buddha Nagar,
21st June 2018.

Vidya Sagar Verma
Former Ambassador of India to Kazakhstan

Transliteration Key

(Sanskrit Text in Devanagari Script in Annexture)

अ = *A*
आ = *Ā*
इ = *I*
ई = *I*
उ = *U*
ऊ = *ū*
ए = *E*
ऐ = *Ai*
ओ = *o / Au*
औ = *Ou*
ऋ = *Ri*
अं (अनुस्वार)= *N/M*
अः (विसर्ग)= *H*

क् = *K*
क = *KA*
ख् = *KH*
ख = *KHA*
ग् = *G*
घ् = *GH*
ङ् = *N*
च् = *CH*
छ् = *CHH*
ज् = *J*
झ् = *JH*
ञ् = *NY*

ट् = *T*
ठ् = *TH*
ड् = *D*
ढ् = *DH*
ण् = *Ń*
त् = *T*
थ् = *TH*
द् = *D*
ध् = *DH*
न् = *N*

प् = *P*
फ् = *F*
ब् = *B*
भ् = *BH*
म् = *M*
य् = *Y*
र् = *R*
ल् = *L*
व् = *V*
श् = *SH*
ष् = *Ś*
स् = *S*
ह् = *H*
क्ष् = *Kś*
त्र् = *TR*
ज्ञ् = *JN*

Contents

Prayer 7
In Praise of God 9
The Divine Promise 10
Message 11
Foreword 13
Preface 15
Transliteration Key 18

Section I

Vedic Philosophy in Diagram 27
1. Introduction to the Philosophy of Yoga 29
2. Yoga: The Science of Mind 30
3. The Purpose of Yoga 33
4. The Universality of Yoga 35
5. Misconceptions about Yoga 37
6. The Constituents of Yoga 39
7. Step I: Moral Discipline 42
8. Step II: Asana (Physical Exercises) 45
9. Step III: *Pranayama* (Breathing Exercises) 46
10. Step IV: Meditation 49
11. What is Meditation? 50
12. Meditation: Revelation of Secrets of Nature 52
13. Meditation: Source of Supernatural Powers 53
14. Experiences in the Hour of Meditation (*Anubhuti*) 56
15. Meditation: Way to Realisation of Self and God 59

Section II

16. The Fundamentals of Ancient Indian Philosophy 67
17. Proofs of Existence of God 69
18. Nature, Attributes and Functions of God 78
19. Nature and Activities of Soul (JIVA) 82
20. Is Time of Death Pre-determined? 86
21. Where is the Soul Located in the Body? 87
22. Relationship between God and Soul 89
23. God and Souls – Entirely Different Entities 92
24. What is Nature (*Prakriti*) and Its Role 95
25. The Doctrine of *Maya* (Illusion) 98
26. The Concept of *Trividha* (Three-fold) *Brahma* 101
27. The Doctrine of *Karma* 104
28. The Gita's Views on *Karma, Akarma, Vikarma* 107
29. *Karma* and Destiny (*Bhgaya*) 109
30. Non-Hindu Sciptures' and Philosophers' Views on *Karma* 113
31. The Doctrine of Reincarnation of Soul 115
32. Proofs of Soul's Reincarnation 117
33. Views of Renowned Philosophers on Reincarnation of Soul 122
34. References of Reincarnation in Non-Hindu Religions 126
35. The Doctrine of *Moksha* (Liberation) 129
36. Is *Moksha* an Eternal State? 133
37. Belief in Return from Liberated State (*Moksha*) in Non-Hindu Cultures 136
38. Yoga – The Workshop of Indian Culture and Philosophy 137
39. Arise! Awake! 139

Section III

40. Practical Lessons in Yoga 147
Photographs of Asanas 150

Step I: Moral Discipline

41. Moral Conduct 163

42. Treat Others Like Thyself 164
43. Follow the Dictates of Your Conscience 166
44. Think about the Opposite or Adverse Consequences 168
45. Be Always Mindful of Death and God 170
46. Inculcate Feelings of Detachment 172
47. Self-Introspection (*ÃTMA – NIRÎKŠAÑ*) 174
48. Complete Control over Senses (*Pratyãhãr*) 176

Step II: *Asana* (Physical Exercises)

49. Instructions Regarding *Asana* and Health 179
50. Meditation-Related *Asanas* 182
51. Health-Related *Asanas* 184
52. *Dhanur Asana* (Bow Posture) 186
53. *Bhujanga Asana* (Cobra Posture) 187
54. *Pashchimottan Asana* (Forward- Bending Posture) 188
55. *Matsya Asana* (Fish Posture) 189
56. *Ardhamatsyendra Asana* (Spinal Twist Posture) 190
57. *Gomukh Asana* (Cow-Head Posture) 191
58. *Makar Asana* (Crocodile Posture) 192
59. *Sarvãnga Asana* (All-Limbs Posture) 193
60. *Hala Asana* (Plough Posture) 194
61. *Shîrša-Asana* (Head Posture) 195
62. *Surya* (*Isha*) *Namaskar Asana* (Salutation to God) 196
63. *Šatkarma* (Six Procedures) 199

Step III: *Prãñãyãma* (Breathing Exercises)

64. Instructions Regarding *Pranayama*: 203
65. Meditation-Related *Trividha Pranayama* 206
66. Meditation-Related *Chathurtha* (Fourth) *Pranayama* 208
67. Health-Related *Svar Parivartan* (Altering Breath) *Nadi Shodan* (Cleansing of Nerves)/*Anulom Vilom Pranayama* 210

68. Health-Related *Svar Parivartan Pranayama* (Altering Breath): *Sûrya Bhedi/Chandra Bhedi Pranayama* 212
69. *Trideshi Pranayama* (Three-Stage Breathing) 213
70. *Bhastrika* (Bellow Breathing) 215
71. *Ujayyî Pranayama* (Throat- Massaging *Pranayama*) 216
72. *Shîtali/Shîtkari Pranayama* (Cooling Exercise) 217
73. *Kapãl Bhãti* (Head-Glow *Pranayama*) 218
74. *Bhrãmari* (Bumble Bee) *Pranayama* 219
75. Synchronised Breathing – *Pranic* Healing (*Tãrtamay Pranayama*) 220

Step IV: Meditation

76. Important Observations regarding Meditation 225
77. *Trãtaka* : Open-Eyed Concentration 227
78. Meditation by Concentration on the Breath 229
79. Meditation by Concentration on Your Forehead (*Ãgya Chakra*) 230
80. Meditation by Concentration on Navel *Chakra* 231
81. Meditation by Recitation of a *Mantra* or Hymn or *Ayat* 232
82. Meditation by Concentration on Objects of Nature 233
83. Meditation by Concentration on Sound (*Anãhat Nãda*) 234
84. Meditation on Eight *Chakrãs* 236
85. Meditation on Any Object of Liking 238
86. Therapeutic Meditation 241
87. Self-Confidence– Related Meditation 243
88. Contemplative Prayer Healing 246
89. Total Devotion to God – *Ishvara Pranidhana* (Does God Listen to One's Prayers?) 248
90. Experiences (*Anubhûti*) During Meditation 251

Annexture 253
मूल संस्कृत उद्धरण
(Sanskrit Text in Devanagari Script)

Section I

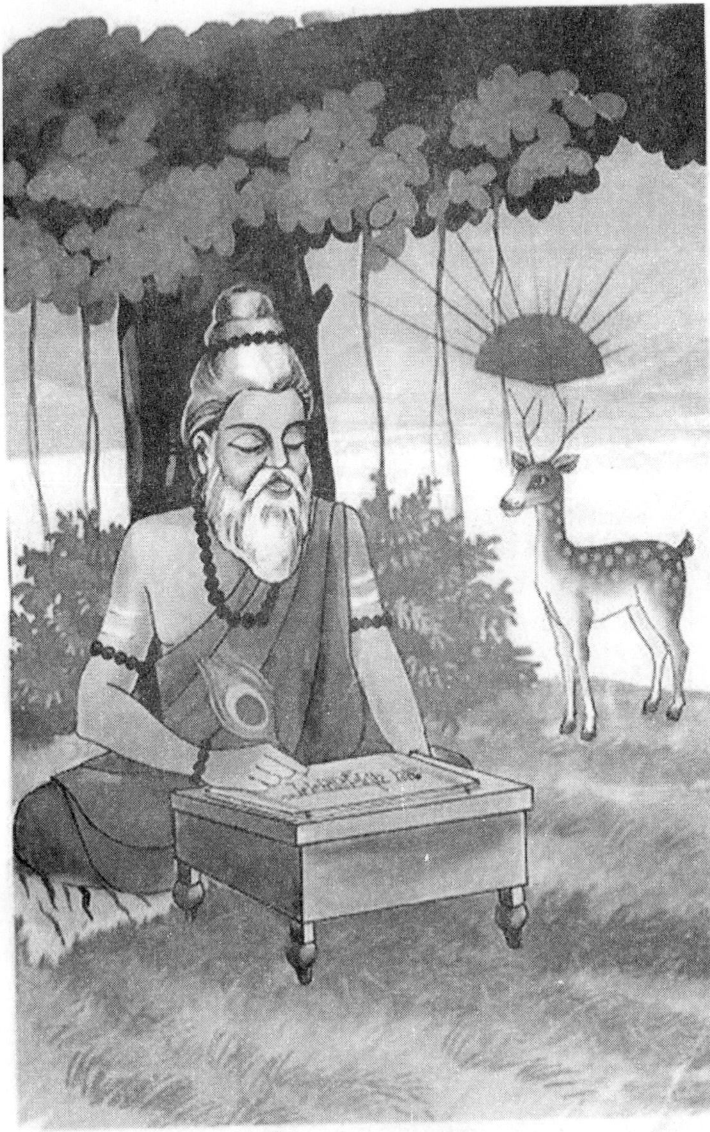

अथ योगानुशासनम्

अब आरम्भ है योग की पद्धति

Now begins the Yoga Discipline

Vedic Nectar

SAHASRÀÑY-AYAM VIYATAU ASYA PAKŠAU
HARER HANSASYA PATATAH SVARGAM
SA DEVÀN SARVÀN URASYA-UPAPADYA
SAMPASHYAN YÀTI BHUVAÑANI VISHVÀ (6)

—Atharva Veda (10.8.18)

Thousands of eons have passed
Our Soul, the Swan, with feathers stretched.
Is flying in search of bliss Divine
All divine powers rest in its heart.
Yet having visited the Universe diverse
Continues flying in search of Bliss.

Vedic Philosophy in Diagram

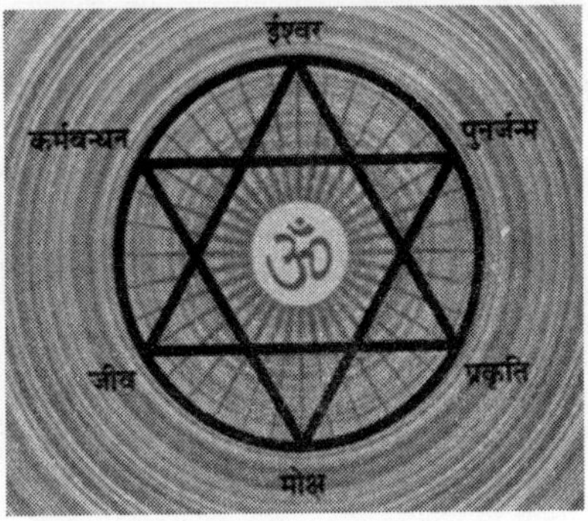

The above circle contains two triangles representing
The Trinity of God, Soul and Nature (Trividha Brahma)
The Triad of Bondage of Action, Reincarnation and Liberation.
The waves emitting from Aum represent the Cosmic Background Radiation at the time of creation.
The circle 'Vritta' represents 'Rita' – Eternal Cosmic Order.

"Throughout and everywhere the true symbol of Nature is the circle, because it is the scheme or type of recurrence."

—Wallace

"In all of us, there dwells a secret marvellous power of freeing ourselves from the changes of time, of withdrawing to our secret selves away from external things, and of so discovering to ourselves the eternal in us in the form of unchangeability. At that time, the external world is no longer an object for us, but is lost in us."

—Schelling

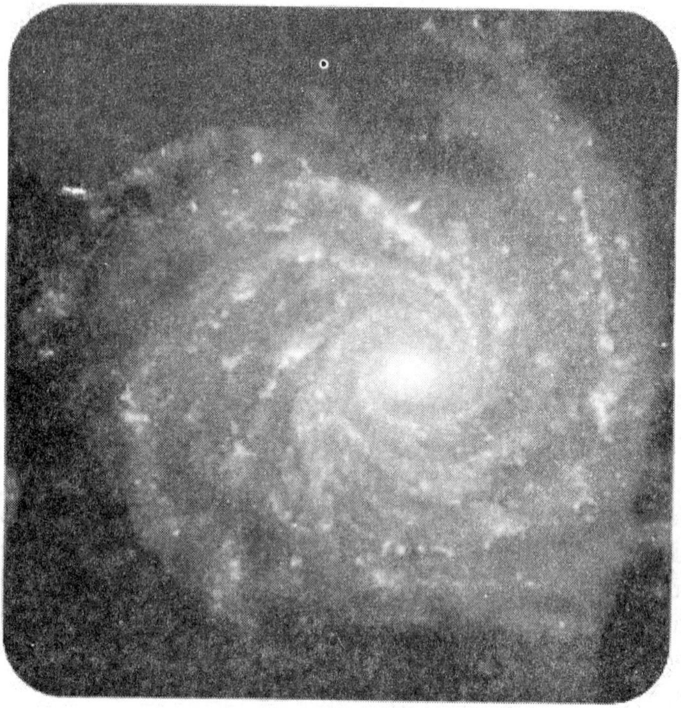

तमेव भान्तमनुभातिसर्वं तस्य भासा सर्वमिदं विभाति

-कठोपनिषद् (2.2.15)

(उसी के प्रकाश से ये सब प्रकाशित होते हैं।
उसकी ज्योति से यह सारा जगत् ज्योतिष्मान होता है।)

अल्लाहो बे कुल्ले शमीन मुहित
अल्लाहो नूर उस समावाति वलअर्द। - कुरान शरीफ़

(Allah surroundeth and encloseth all
His light illumineth all heaven and earth)

– The Holy Quran

God said let there be light and there was light.
– The Holy Bible (Genesis 1.3)

सरब जोतिमहिं जाकि जोत। - गुरुग्रन्थसाहिब

1
Introduction to the Philosophy of Yoga

Yoga is an ancient spiritual discipline which finds mention in the Vedas which are universally acknowledged as the oldest books in the Library of Mankind. The Yoga discipline is also described in the Upanishads about which German philosopher Schopenhauer had stated, "In the whole world, there is no study so beneficial and so elevating as that of the Upanishads. It has been the solace of my life – it will be solace at my death." In fact, in all the ancient scriptures of India, Yoga finds an honoured place.

The philosophy of Yoga is found in the old scriptures like jewels scattered all over the field. It is, however, Sage Patanjali who over 3,000 years back put the Yoga philosophy in a systematic treatise called 'Yoga *Darshana*'. The treatise is in Sutras (Aphorisms). It is, therefore, also called Yoga *Sutra*. His philosophy of Yoga is known as Ashtanga Yoga (Eight-Part-Yoga).

The Yoga Effect

NA TASYA ROGO NA JARÃ NA MRITYUH
PRÃPTASYA YOGA-AGNIM AYAM SHRÎRAM (121),

One whose body has been castigated by the heat of Yoga,
Suffers from neither Disease nor Oldage nor Death.
—Shvetashvatar Upanishad (2.12)

2
Yoga: The Science of Mind

The subject matter of Yoga is Mind. Yoga is rightly called the Science of Mind. Sage Patanjali states: 'YOGAH CHITTAVRITTI NIRODHAH' (7): "Controlling the thought currents of Mind is Yoga." (This aphorism appears on the cover page of this book also). '*Vrittis*' are the thought currents or modifications or activities of the Mind. When Yoga is all about Mind, let us know what is Mind and what are its functions.

Once a disciple asked Swami Shivanada, "Who is the greatest enemy of man?" The Swami replied, "Mind." Strange, but true, because all the baser instincts are the products of mind. Jealousy, hatred, greed, lust, anger, vengeance are all the products of one's mind. When one is overpowered by these instincts, all sorts of crimes and sins like theft, murder, rape are committed. Thus, mind becomes the cause of bondage and, thereby, sufferings.

It is also true, if Swami Shivananda were asked who is the greatest friend of man, the Swami would have replied again "Mind." Surprised? Mind is our greatest friend because all the good actions, all the spiritual and material progress, all the discoveries and inventions can be made only by the mind. Thus, Mind is also the source of happiness. In the Indian scriptures, it is stated: MANA EVA MANUŠYÃNÃM KÃRAÑAM BANDHA MOKŠAYOH (8), i.e., Mind is the cause of bondage as also the cause of liberation. The same idea has been expressed by John Milton in his epic 'The Paradise Lost' thus:

"The Mind in its own place and in itself,
Can make a heav'n of hell, a hell of heav'n."

This all depends on how we use our mind. It is just like a knife which, if we use with care, can be helpful in cutting vegetables and fruits; if we use it carelessly, we may cut our fingers.

Mind is a powerful agent bestowed by Nature to us. It has a vast potential. Psychologists tell us that we use only 10% of the capacity of our brain which is controlled by mind. The unused 90% can be opened up to us by the Yogic way, Meditation.

Mind is working all the time, non-stop. Even when we are asleep, our mind is functioning by way of having dreams. Mind can think of only one thing at a time. Sometimes it happens when we are listening, but still not registering anything; we are seeing but still not seeing. It is because our mind is preoccupied with some other thing. Most of the time we are not aware about its functioning. Such a situation is called absent-mindedness. A child is reading a book, but not understanding a line, because his mind is in the play-field. We are sitting at the dining table with our family members, but engrossed in the problems of the office. Our mind is not at the dining table. That is why, such a situation is called absent-mindedness. Often, we are thinking, but not thinking about the thing or subject we want to think. The Yoga teaches us the technique to control our thought processes, to channelise our thinking by paying undivided attention to the subject we want to think. When this happens, full knowledge about the thing or subject dawns on us.

Now, who is to use or control the Mind? Spirit, Soul. While the modern psychology and western philosophy treat Mind as conscious, the Indian scriptures regard Mind as just a product of matter. Mind is just an adjunct of the Soul, its instrument. Swami Vivekananda has succinctly described Mind in the following words: "Mind at a very low rate of vibration is what is known as matter. Matter at the high rate of vibration is what is known as mind. Both are the same substance."

If Mind is not conscious, how does it appear conscious? Mind attains consciousness from the Soul in the same manner as the Moon gets illumined by the rays of the Sun, or as a piece of iron gets magnetised in contact with a piece of magnet. Similarly, all our deeds appear to be performed by the mind, but behind the mind is the Soul which spurs all action. Mind being a product of matter cannot act on its own. Perhaps an analogy of artificial intelligence can make this idea clear. A computer with artificial intelligence makes intelligent processing or a robot undertakes fantastic tasks but the real 'actor' is the Software Engineer who devises and installs the relevant software. It is also equally true that Soul cannot act when it is not in a body. It always acts through the agency of mind. Renowned Sanskrit poet Kalidasa has stated: SHARÎRAM ADYA KHALU DHARMA SÃDHANAM (9), i.e., Verily, our body is the instrument of righteous deeds. The Bible also states:

"The Temple of God is holy and you are that Temple,". Meaning thereby that we can worship God only through our body. Here comes the role of Yoga, viz., controlling and channelising the thought currents of mind in the right direction.

Thus Spake Bulle Shâh

O BULIA! RAB DÃ KÎ PÃÑÃ
ITHO PUTÑÃ TE ITHE LÃÑÃ

O Bulia! What is realisation of God?
It is uprooting Mind from here
(Worldly attachments)
And transplanting it here
(in spirituality/dedication to God)

3
The Purpose of Yoga

Every human being possesses three things – Body, Mind and Soul (Spirit).

The purpose of Yoga is physical, mental and spiritual development. In ancient Indian philosophy, of which Yoga is the core, the summum bonum of life is the union of Soul with God. And Yoga is the only way to achieve it. The literal meaning of the word 'Yoga' is union (its English equivalent is Yoke, to Join). That is why, Yoga has been defined as: SAMYOGO YOGA ITY UKTO JIVÃTMA-PARAMÃTMANORITI (10), i.e., Yoga is the union of Soul and God. The Vedas and the Upanishads advise 'ÃTMÃNAM VIDHI' (11), i.e., Know Thyself. Same is the command of The Holy Bible.

The Vedas also declare: AMRITASYA PUTRÃH (4), i.e., You are the children of the Immortal (God). The Holy Bible (Psalm 82.6) expresses the same sentiment: "I have said ye are gods, and all of you are children of the Most High." The Holy Quran also says the same thing: LA ILAHA ILA ANNA, i.e., there is no god, I am the god. The propose of quoting these holy texts is to remind ourselves that there is a Divine Spark in all of us and that, because of ignorance, we are not aware of it and, hence, the advice to know ourselves. And that can be done only through Yoga by chiselling that Divine Spark. God being present everywhere is present in our Souls too and can be discerned there directly. In this context, the following words of a few renowned philosophers will help us understand the purpose of Yoga:

1. The Soul in this profundity has a likeness and an affable nearness to God.... In this deepest, most inner and most secret depth of the Soul, God essentially, really and substantially exists.

—Tauler

2. The purpose of Yoga is to unite man with the Divine Ground, with the Cosmic Consciousness. Yoga is the psychological linking of the mind to the super-ordinated principal 'by which the mind knows'.

—Allie M. Frazier

3. Meditation is the way to knowing and beholding the eternal, indestructible, essential centre of our being.

—Rudolf Steiner

4. Contemplation and vision of God is Man's absolute good.

—St. Thomas Aquinas

While Yoga is essentially a spiritual pursuit, it is not closed to those who do not believe in Soul or God. For such agnostics as also for the lay, the Gita offers a secular definition of Yoga, viz., YOGAH KARMASU KAUSHALAM, i.e., Yoga is perfection in action. By controlling the thought currents of one's mind, one attains deep concentration on any subject matter and, thereby, attains complete knowledge of the matter pondered over. This adds to attaining perfection in action. Many discoveries of science have been made by deep contemplation. Stephen Hawking observes, "Newton has said that the idea of gravity came to him as he sat in contemplative mood and was occasioned by the fall of an apple."

Thus Spake Albert Einstein

My religion consists of a humble admiration of the illimitable, superior spirit who reveals Himself in the slight details, we are able to perceive with our frail and feeble mind.

4
The Universality of Yoga

Whether one believes in the existence of God, Soul, Reincarnation or not is a matter of faith. Even those who do not believe in these matters, the Yoga Discipline is open to them. The Yoga has a universal appeal. Yoga is of two types – the Spiritual Yoga and the Secular Yoga. If you believe in God, Soul, Reincarnation et al will be helpful for practising Spiritual Yoga. However, those who do not believe in the existence of God or Soul or Reincarnation, need not desert Yoga on that account. Just as the Sun shines equally on the theists and the atheists or water quenches thirst of all beings, so does the discipline of Yoga benefit all practitioners. All the same, just as the Sun or Water is to be approached in a specific way to tap solar or hydro-energy, the discipline of Yoga releases extraordinary powers to the practitioners who follow the prescribed procedure. Those who meditate on the spiritual aspect of Yoga, advance spiritually, as did Swami Dayananda Saraswati, Swami Vivekanada and Yogi Auribindo Ghose. Those who meditate on secular matters like the objects of Nature, are enlightened about the material matters as did Newton discover the Law of Gravity.

The discipline of Yoga develops an individual physically, mentally and spiritually. All human beings are alike, so the system of Yoga is equally beneficial to all, irrespective of religion or nationality. A person born in the cold climate of Siberia where temperature reaches –50 degrees Celsius and a person born in the hot climate of Sahara Desert where temperature reaches +50 degrees Celsius, both have the same body temperature at 37 degrees Celsius. Similarly, while in anger, blood pressure goes up, heart beat and breath rate increase in all the human beings, whether they belong to India or Australia, Asia or Africa. As the system of Yoga deals with body, mind and Soul, it will benefit equally everybody. In other words, Yoga is not an exclusive discipline for Indians or Hindus, it is for the whole human race.

Studies have been conducted in the West and it has been established by scientific researches that the system of Yoga is beneficial for the composite development of human personality. Yoga provides deep rest and relaxation. Physiological experiments provided evidence that through the regular practice of meditation, causes of hypertension, anxiety, high blood pressure, cardiac arrest and other psychosomatic illnesses are removed. Yoga lessons have been found beneficial to students who were drug addicts. Their relations with fellow students, teachers and parents improved and they stopped taking drugs. Noting such beneficial effects, the General Assembly of the State of Illinois passed a resolution (No. 677 on 24.5.1972) recommending lessons in meditation in academic institutions. Noted Yoga master Luis S.R. Vas has commented: "Meditation is an ancient religious practice being routinely prescribed in modern society, not just by spiritual masters, but by behavioural scientists, medical practitioners and business consultants." Consequently, a good number of Yoga centres have come up in the West which conduct Yoga courses for highly placed businessmen, high officials of Government departments. It is found that such persons with onerous responsibilities experienced lesser tension, greater productivity and better inter-personal relations and improved professional proficiency.

The Universality of Yoga has been acknowledged by the United Nations General Assembly in their unanimous resolution in December 2014, declaring 21st June as International Day of Yoga, which is now being enthusiastically observed all over the world including Pakistan, Bangladesh and Saudi Arabia.

5
Misconceptions about Yoga

There are a few misunderstandings about Yoga. The most common misunderstanding is that only *Asanas* (physical exercises) are the complete Yoga. *Asanas* are only one component of the Yoga system. Its purpose is to keep the body fit and to generate capacity to sit still in one posture, without any movement, for a long duration of time so that one could meditate without distraction. In the whole Yoga *Darshana* of 195 *Sutras* (Aphorisms), only three *Sutras* pertain to *Asanas* and all the three are related to meditation. Similarly, only six *Sutras* pertain to *Pranayama* and these too are in the context of meditation. Most of the prevalent Yoga *Asanas* and *Pranayama* (breathing exercises) pertain to Hatha Yoga and not Patanjali Yoga. These are beneficial for physical fitness but not for meditation, the core of the Yoga system, e.g., one cannot meditate while in *Shirsha Asana* (Head Posture). All the rest of the Yoga *Sutras* pertain to moral discipline and meditation. Without meditation, the *Asanas* are no more than a physical exercise. Rev. Albert Mohler Jr. has succinctly made this point clear: "You may be twisting yourself into pretzels or grasshoppers, but if there is no meditation or direction of consciousness, you are not practising Yoga." – President, Southern Baptist Theosophical Society.

The second misunderstanding is that Yoga is thought to be standing on one leg with both arms raised up for hours together, excessive fasting, or indulging in self-torture in the name of *Tapa*. Tapa means control of senses or undergoing rigorous discipline in spiritual pursuits, e.g., taking a vow to speak the truth or not to harm anyone physically, verbally or mentally, which is not an easy task to undertake.

Third, it is alleged that Yoga teaches Black Magic. This charge is absolutely false. Some practices of the Yoga are misused by some misguided selfish practitioners for fooling people for nefarious gains.

Yoga is a spiritual discipline. It even regards the divine powers called *Siddhis*, achieved during the course of Yoga practice as a hindrance in the path of ultimate goal of Self-realisation or God realisation. How can it endorse such nefarious Black Magic tactics?

Fourth, it is alleged that Yoga teaches us to suppress our senses which is psychologically harmful. Yoga does not teach us to suppress our senses, but to sublimate our senses by changing our thought pattern. The Gita (2.62) says: DHYÃYATO VIŠYÃN PUNSAH SANGASTEŠU UPAJÃYATE (12) i.e. when a man constantly thinks of the objects of sense, attachment to them is produced. The Yoga teaches to divert mind's attention from the sense objects, so no attachment is produced. In the absence of any attachment to sense objects, the question of suppression of senses does not arise. Instead of being attracted towards outward objects, it teaches us how to revel in the inward realities. Dr. S. Radhakrishnan's following words aptly describe this phenomenon: "To hear the melodies of spirit, we must shut off the noise of the world. This is not to renounce the powers of sight, hearing and speech. It is to open the inner eye to the spiritual realities, capture the sounds that come from the world of spirit, sing in silence the hymn of praise to the Supreme Being." (Indian Philosophy).

Fifth, it is also alleged that Yoga teaches us to develop the Self but it ignores the Society. This charge is also baseless. Developing qualities of head and heart like truthfulness, non-violence, non-stealing, non-possessiveness directly contributes to the betterment of the society. The Yoga teaches us to develop our Self so as to encompass the whole humanity to be part of our family. It develops in us the feeling of VASUDHAIVA KUTUMBAKAM (13), i.e., the whole world is a family. The Yoga dose of detachment (towards our relatives) contributes to expansion of our Self to love the whole humanity, as a vaccine develops in us resistance to ward off small pox or other diseases. The following words of Aldous Huxley are pertinent on this issue. "There is good evidence to show that such practices (mediation, self-control) may produce very valuable results. It is possible for a man who employs the methods of mortification or Yoga to achieve a high degree of non-attachment to 'the things of this world' and at the same time, to so heighten his consciousness that he can attach himself more completely than the normal man, to that which is greater than himself, to the integrating principle of all being."

—Aldous Huxley (Ends and Means: Page 233).

6

The Constituents of Yoga

Yoga *Darshana* of Sage Patanjali is in four chapters: *Samãdhi Pãda*, *Sãdhana Pãda*, *Vibhûti Pãda* and *Kaivalya Pãda*. In *Samãdhi Pada*, there is description of *Vrittis*, the modifications or thought currents of mind; mention of methods of controlling these *Vrittis* by *Vairãgya* (Non-Attachment) and *Abhyãsa* (Practice), by *Pranayama* (Breathing Exercises), by *Ishvara Pranidhana* (Dedication to God) or by meditating on any object of one's liking as also Control of the *Vrittis* leading to the state of *Samãdhi* (Trance/ State of Ecstasy). The *Samãdhi* is of two kinds – *Samprajnãt Samadhi* or *Sabija Samãdhi* (containing seeds for future life) and *Asamprajnãt Samãdhi* or *Nirbija Samãdhi* (seedless samadhi) in which all *Vrittis* of mind are extinct and the seeds of new life are burnt out and one breaks the Cycle of Birth and Death. This is called *Kaivalya* or *Moksha* (Liberation/Salvation).

In *Sãdhan Pada*, the ways and means of attaining *Samãdhi* and, thereby, Liberation are described. Liberation, strictly speaking, is liberation from sufferings. In this chapter, there is description of causes of suffering – five *Kleshas* (Afflictions): (i) *Avidya* (Nescience/wrong knowledge/*Mithya Gyan*) mistaking the non-eternal for the eternal, the impure for the pure, the unpleasant for the pleasant and the non-self for the self; (ii) Asmita, i.e., erroneous identification of oneself with the instruments of body and mind; (iii) *Rãga,* i.e., attachment; to pleasant things; (iv) *Dveša,* i.e., hatred of unpleasant things and (v) *Abhinivesha,* i.e., the instinctive love of life and the dread of death. *Chitta* or mind is beset with these afflictions. Deliverance/Liberation consists in severing the relation of Self/Soul and *Chitta* (*Prakriti*). For attaining Liberation/*Moksha*, eight measures are advised in the Yoga *Darshana* (detailed later).

In *Vibhûti Pada*, we find description of *Dhãrana*, *Dhãyãna*, *Samãdhi*. *Dhãrana* is concentration on any object or subject; *Dhãyãna* is contemplation or meditation on the same subject and when the same process of thinking proceeds on the same subject, without extraneous thoughts coming in between, is called *Samadhi*. The process of meditating on the same subject all through *Dhãrana*, *Dhãyãna* and *Samadhi* bears a technical name called *Sanyama*. (However, we have used the word 'Meditation' for it). In *Vibhuti Pada,* there is description of various supernatural powers which a Yogi attains after rigorous *Sadhana*. The accrual of these supernatural powers indicates that the Yogi is on the right path. Sage Patanjali forewarns that indulgence in these powers will obstruct his onward march to attain *Moksha*.

In *Kaivalya Pada*, we learn that ignorance leads us to vicious actions which bind us. Soul's experiences and desires to relive the *Prakriti* – given enjoyments and pleasures generate *Vãsanãs*, which again bind him to the Cycle of Birth and Death. Here we also learn that *Chitta* or mind is the cause of bondage. When *Chitta* is withdrawn from the attractions of *Prakriti*, it goes to sleep and the Soul is released from the clutches of *Prakriti*. The Soul resides in itself. This is the state of *Kaivalya* or *Moksha*. *Kaivalya* literally means 'being alone'. This is also known as Self-Realisation or God-Realisation. (The concepts mentioned in the Yoga *Darshana* are discussed in the subsequent pages).

Sage Patanjali enumerated eight constituents of Yoga, that is why his Yoga system is called *Ashtãnga* Yoga (Eight-Part Yoga). These are *Yama* (Restraints). *Niyama* (Practices), *Ãsana* (Physical Posture), *Prãnayãma* (Breathing Exercises), *Pratyãhãra* (Reversal of Senses – Sublimation of Senses), *Dhãrana* (Concentration), *Dhyãna* (Meditation) and *Samãdhi* (Trance/Ecstasy).

A bit of elaboration of these constituents is necessary. *Yama* means Restraints, controlling one's senses in which they revel. It is sublimation of senses. *Yama* (Restraints) are five: *Ahimsã* (Non-violence), *Satya* (Truthfulness), *Asteya* (Non-stealing/ Honesty), *Brahmacharya* (Control over lust) and *Aparigraha* (Non-possessiveness/non-acquisitiveness). *Niyama* means observance: that which is to be done regularly as a duty. *Niyamas* are also five: *Shauch* (Cleanliness), *Santosha* (Contentment), *Tapa* (Control over Senses), *Svadhyaya* (Study of Scriptures/Self-Introspection) and *Ishvara*

Pranidhãna (Dedication to God). In the state of *Pratyahara*, the mind withdraws from sense objects and sense organs follow the mind in higher pursuits. This is called sublimation of senses.

It needs to be noted that Sage Patanjali has used the word '*Ashtanga*' for the constituents of Yoga. '*Ashta*' means eight and '*Anga*' means organ/limb (part of the body). As in a body all the organs are important, so is in the case of Yoga. Even if the head is the most important part of the body, if any other part is missing or dysfunctional, one is considered handicapped. Similarly, even though *Samadhi* is the most important part of Yoga system, the other parts, e.g., *Yama*, *Niyama* are equally important. Otherwise one cannot make desired progress in the Yoga practice. All the parts of Yoga can be practised simultaneously as do all parts of body function in harmony.

For the sake of simplification and better understanding, we have put all these eight constituents in Four Steps. *Yama*, *Niyama* and *Pratyahara* are under Step 1: Moral Discipline. *Asana* is under Step II: Physical Exercises. *Pranayama* is under Step III: Breathing Exercises. The last three – *Dhãrana*, *Dhyãna* and *Samadhi* are under Step IV: Meditation. Nothing has been left out, only re-categorised for better comprehension and greater felicity. All the constituents are explained below.

Thus Spake Alfred Noyes

How shall I find It? Only through those doors
Which, opening inward, in each separate soul
Give each man access to that soul of all
Living within each life, not to be found
Or known, till looking inward each alone
Meets the unkowleable and eternal God.

7
Step I: Moral Discipline

Yoga is a spiritual way of life. Moral Discipline is an integral part of it. Without advancement in this aspect of Yoga, progress in other aspects will be difficult. Even if one does not believe in God or Soul, one will have to follow this discipline. The moral discipline is not only essential for the fabric of the society, it is essential for one's own well-being also. If one is beset with anger, hatred, jealously, greed or lust, can he compose himself and sit in meditation? One has to control these baser emotions and inculcate qualities like compassion, truthfulness, helpfulness, contentment, and love for humanity. It will be seen what is taught in Moral Discipline is nothing new. These are normal ethical and human values which are taught in every religion. Sage Patanjali advises us to be ethically alert, e.g., theft is not just stealing. *Asteya* (Non-Stealing) is honest living. Non-payment of Government taxes is theft; accepting bribes or favours for what is done in one's official capacity is theft; not doing one's office work or slipping away from office is also theft. Only physical assault is not violence. *Ahimsa* (Non-Violence) comprises not to kill any being, e.g., for meat eating; not to harass anybody mentally, verbally or harm anybody financially. Similarly, *Satya* (Truth) is a comprehensive concept. It comprises the whole gamut of moral and spiritual order. One should always act truthfully, verbally, mentally, financially and socially. Truthfulness makes a person pious. In fact, nothing in the world can work if truth is ignored. William Blake said:

"If the Sun and the Moon should doubt,
They will immediately go out."

Santosha (Contentment) is not merely to be contented with material possessions. While competition is good, overweening ambition, in which one loses one's calm or balance and harms others to get promotion is reflection of discontentment. This leads to tension, high blood pressure and heart attack. One has to inculcate high moral sense in oneself, otherwise one will not be able to get peace of mind which is the real purpose of Yoga. And this can be done by oneself alone.

Sage Pantajali has prescribed a few more measures for one's spiritual elevation. One, *Svãdhyãya,* i.e., study of scriptures and other good literature and self-introspection. Good ideas lead to good actions and while introspecting how many good ideas you have inculcated in your lifestyle, you become more and more spiritual. Mark Twain had advised, "The man who does not read good books has no advantage over the one who cannot read." Two, *Aparigraha* (Non-Possessiveness). Ordinary man is self-centred and is always engrossed in amassing things for himself and his family contributing to plunder of Nature's resources. Vishnu Purana says: Even if all the pleasures and desirable things in the world are made available to one person, he cannot feel contented or happy because the source of happiness does not lie in material things, but in God. Therefore, Sage Patanjali has advised non-acquisitiveness. Arthur Schopenhaur has also advised, "Wealth is like sea water; the more we drink, the thirstier we become." Three, *Ishvara Pranidhan* (Devotion to God). *Ishvara Pranidhan* is that state of mind when one forgets about oneself, devotes oneself to the service of humanity and surrenders oneself to the will of God. He is in the state of mind like that of a lost child in a fair where no amount of beautiful toys and delicious foods please him and is always crying to meet his mother. This is a high state of spiritual elevation which leads him to attain *Samadhi*.

Sage Patanjali has not only spelt out the core values for spiritual elevation, as a great 'Physician of the Mind', he is also aware that it is not that easy to follow these values in real life where there are many temptations and other situations when one is swept off one's feet and follows the opposite. For such a situation, the Sage advises: VITARKA BÃDHANE PRATIPAKŠA BHÃVANAM (14) (Yoga Darshana – II.33), i.e., when the mind is swayed by evil thoughts, constant pondering over the results of these thoughts, if enacted, is the remedy, e.g., when tempted to take bribe or make adulteration in foodstuff or medicines, one may mentally visualise oneself being caught and being put in jail. Such a counter-thought will invoke fear in him and he will desist from doing this.

Path to spirituality has to be worked out by oneself and the following words of Swami Vivekananda are the guiding principle:

"You have to grow from the inside out. None can teach you, None can make you spiritual. There is no other teacher, but your own Soul."

Once your Soul becomes alert, you are saved from the wrong-doings, the cause of suffering. Rudyard Kipling assures us: "If your being is right, your doing cannot possibly go wrong."

Thus Spake Manu on Dharma

Dhritih Kšamâ Damo Asteyam
Shaucham Indriya-Nigrhâ
Dhîr Vidyâ Satyam Akrodho
Dhashkam Dharma Lakšañam

—Manusmṛiti 6.92

Pateince, Pardon, Control over Mind, Non-Stealing, Cleanliness of Mind and Body, Control over Senses, Wisdom, Right Knowledge, Truth and Control over Anger are the ten traits or constituents of Dharma ie moral conduct.

8

Step II: Asana (Physical Exercises)

'*Asana*' means to be seated. It is often translated as physical posture. Asana in the Yoga system has dual purpose: (i) to keep your body fit; and (ii) to be able to sit in a stable, comfortable position for a long duration of time, without any movement, so that one can meditate without disturbance. Asanas also help you in warding off thirst and hunger, heat and cold during meditation.

Sage Patanjali defines Asana: STHIRA - SUKHAM - ÃSANAM (15), i.e., 'Asana' means sitting still in a comfortable posture for meditation. St. Augustine has rightly commented, "The comfort of our posture has much to do with the continuous stream of our meditation." Cross-legged posture is very comfortable for meditation for a majority of practitioners.

Sitting stable without movement for a long duration of time requires the body to be absolutely fit. For physical fitness, there are numerous Asanas propounded by Hatha Yoga, mostly named after postures of birds and animals. These Asanas are geared to tone up different parts of body. The diseases which inflict us often relate to digestive system, respiratory system, blood circulatory system or spinal cord, which is the main channel of the control of the nervous system. Other problems relate to the mind. Particular Asanas are suitable for warding off particular diseases. In the Practical Lessons, the methods of doing a few Asanas have been indicated alongwith their benefits.

As *Asanas* have visual impact, the Asana component of Yoga often gets more publicity than it deserves. It is often projected as a complete Yoga, which it is not. Asana is a preliminary constituent of Yoga discipline.

9
Step III: *Pranayama* (Breathing Exercises)

Pranayama is a very important part of the Yoga discipline. '*Prana*' means vital energy, which is its subtle form. *Prana's* outer form is breath, air. Its significance can be judged from the fact that we can live without food for two weeks or so; we can live without water for two days or so; but we cannot live without breathing even for a single minute.

We know when we breathe in, we inhale oxygen. Oxygen purifies our blood; helps in digestion; cleans up the respiratory system and removes toxins of the body when we breathe out. That is why, the breath which comes out is foul. The Rig Veda (10.137.2) describes the function of *Prana* thus:

DVÃVIMAU VÃTAU VÃTA Ã SINGHORÃ PRÃVATAH
DAKŠAM TE ANYA Ã VÃTU PARÃNYO VÃTU YADRAPAH (16)

i.e., in the body, two types of Air (*Prana*) flow – Inhalation and Exhalation. One of them flows to the Ocean (Heart) and the other to the outer environment. The one brings with it health and vitality, the other takes away foul smell and diseases. Here the heart is likened to an ocean, because it receives impure blood through the veins like rivers flow into the ocean. Just as the water is purified through the sun rays and pours down (rains) as fresh water, similarly, heart purifies the blood and sends forth clean blood to the body through the arteries.

Breathing exercises also help us in improving concentration. There is a saying: "CHALE VÃTE CHALAM CHITTAM NISHCHALE NISHCHALO BHAVET (17), i.e., when *Prana* moves, Mind moves; when *Prana* is steadied, Mind becomes steady. That is why, when you want to take a photograph you are advised to hold your breath before clicking the camera. If you have better concentration, your memory gets sharpened and your intellect becomes more analytical. Greater flow of oxygen through *Pranayama* into the brain improves its overall functioning of the body.

Prana also controls our emotions. It is a psychological fact that our breath rate increases when we are angry. When angry, if you take three deep breaths, anger will cool down. All our emotions have different breath rates. This shows that breathing exercises help in controlling emotions. Manusmriti says: Just as the dross of metals is burnt up by heating it up, the dross of the senses is removed through *Pranayama*, which sublimates the senses.

Apart from concentration, cleansing the body system and controlling emotions, *Pranayama* provides vitality to our body. *Prana* is called vitality. The *Hatha* Yoga has propounded some breathing exercises which are very helpful for removing diseases and providing energy to the body. We can see, the flow of energy in karate exercises. A karate expert is a person like you and me and eats the same food as we do. Where from he gets energy that he can break bricks with a stroke of his hand? He regulates his breath in such a manner that he concentrates energy in a particular part of the body, e.g., hand or leg and releases the energy with a stroke. Similarly, you would have seen trucks plying at high speed on the roads carrying tonnes of weight. But if a tyre of such a truck gets deflated, it cannot move even a few metres. If it does, its wheel will be twisted and tyre will be torn. It is obvious, the weight is carried by the air inside the tyre and not by the wheel. Furthermore, a storm uproots huge trees and blows away with it whatever comes in its way. Where from the storm, the wind, gets strength? It is *Prana*. Our scriptures say: PRÃÑÃD VÃYUR AJÃYATA (18), i.e., Wind is born of *Prana*. This shows *Prana*, of which wind is only the outer manifestation, provides strength. Brihidãrañyaka Upanishad states: PRÃÑO VAI BALAM TAT PRÃÑE PRATIŠTHITAM (19), i.e., Prana is energy; that energy is established in *Prana*.

Prana is said to have three *Vrittis*, i.e., tendancies. *Taitreya Ãranyaka* says: TRIVRID VAI PRÃÑÃH (20), i.e., *Prana* has three tendencies. Yoga *Darshana* names them as *Bãhya Vritti* (Exhalation), *Abhyantara Vritti* (Inhalation) and *Stambha Vritti* (Retention), holding the *Prana* where it is. This is also called *Kumbhaka Vritti*. Yoga

Darshana also mentions fourth *Vritti* as BÃHYA – ABHYÃNTARA – VIŠAYA – ÃKŠEPI –CHATURTHAH (21), i.e., interrupting the two-way flow of *Prana* is the Fcurth *Pranayama*. This must be clarified here that all the four aforesaid *Pranayamas* (Breathing Exercises) are for meditation purposes. This section also contains *Hatha* Yoga *Pranayama* (Breathing Exercise is) which helpful for physical fitness and removal of diseases, although these are not part of the Patanjali Yoga *Darshana*. (Their method is given in Section III, Step II: Breathing Exercises).

Thus Spake Sâdî

Each breath that goeth in, strengthens the life;
Each that comes out, the body purifies;
Each breathing in and – out, two blessings bring;
Then think of Him with each, with two-fold thanks

10
Step IV: Meditation

Having purged oneself of the baser instincts, having developed capacity to sit steadily and comfortably for a long duration of time, having learnt the art of controlling the breathing process and havng trained one's senses to look inward and follow the direction of the mind, one qualifies to practise the core of Yoga, the meditative process. Meditation ie Samâdhi is the apex of Yoga discipline. English equivalent of Smadhi is Trance or Ecstatic State. It is the gateway to liberation, Self-Realisation and God-Realisation.

Thus Spake Plotinus On Trance

The Soul is no longer conscious of the body or of the mind,
but knows that she has what she desired,
that she is where no deception can come,
and that she would not exchange her bliss
for all the heaven of heavens.

11
What is Meditation?

Meditation comprises *Dhãrana* (Concentration/Retention), *Dhãyãna* (Contemplation) and *Samadhi* (Trance/Ecstatic State). The three taken together bear the technical name *Sanyama*. *Dhãrana* is to retain in the mind an object or subject, which could be internal or external and not to let it slip away, and if it does, to mentally catch it and bring it back again within its ambit. The object of retention or concentration could be internal like navel, heart, forehead, or external like the sun, any heavenly body or a flower. But the mind must remain focussed on it all the time, without any obstruction or diversion. After some time, this *Dhãrana* passes into *Dhãyãna*.

Dhãyãna is contemplation on the same object or subject of *Dhãrana*, without allowing any extraneous thoughts to intervene. It is channelising the uninterrupted flow of thought in one direction like the flow of water from a tap. In this stage, no other thoughts should come to one's mind except the thoughts related to the thing or subject thought about. The steady flow of *Dhyãna* passes into *Samadhi*.

In *Dhãyãna* one is aware of oneself, of the object of thought and the thinking process. But in *Samadhi*, the *Dhyãta* (Knower), the *Dhyãna* (Knowning) and the *Dhyeya* (the object thought about) all merge into one. It is as if one forgets oneself and only the object thought about illuminates and the Knower knows all aspects of it in entirety. This State is likened to a crystal-ball which becomes red in the presence of a red object and appears to lose its colourlessness.

One thing is to be borne in mind that *Dhãrãna*, *Dhyãna* and *Samadhi* are a continuous process of thinking with regard to the same object or subject. It is not possible to have *Dhãrana* on one subject and *Dhyãna* on another subject and *Samadhi* still on another subject.

No, all are one continuous process. As all are to be executed together, Sage Patanjali has given a technical term '*Sanyama*' for all the three as a composite whole. (We have, however, used the word 'Meditation' for *Sanyama*). Just as the same water of the Ganga flows uninterrupted in Gangotri, Haridwar and Kashi and other rivulets merging on the way, if the similar flow of thought runs through *Dhãrana*, *Dhyãna* and *Samadhi* and other identical (*Sajãtiya*) thoughts pouring in, Yogi is performing *Sanyama*.

Now what is the outcome (Fruit) of the state of *Sanyama*? Sage Patanjali says: TAJJAYÃT PRAJNÃ-ÃLOKAH (22), i.e., On mastering of it, descends the light of intellectual consciousness that illumines all the aspects of the object/subject thought about. This has been called '*Ritambharã Prajnã*' in *Samadhi Pada*. This is that intuitive faculty of mind in which Yogi discerns the Eternal Cosmic Order and the Eternal Moral and Spiritual Order. Now the Yogi sees the things in their true state as they are (*Yathãrtha Svarup*). He now sees, as it were, the Mind of God, to use the term of Stephen Hawking.

We have mentioned earlier that *Samadhi* is of two types – *Samprajnãta* or Conscious and *Asamprajnãta* or Superconscious. *Samprajnãta* is called *Sabija* (with seed) *Samadhi* and *Asamprajnãta* is called *Nirbija* (Seedless) *Samadhi*. In *Sabija Samadhi*, one is meditating on an object, and passing through the stages of deliberation (*Vitarka*), reflection (*Vichãra*), joy (*Ananda*) and sense of personality (*Asmita*). These are forms of concentration which have definite object on which they rest. These are called *Avalamban*, i.e., Prop or Support. *Samprajnãta* or *Sabija Samadhi* is a state of *Ekãgrata* (Concetration) and *Asamprajnãta* or *Nirbija Samadhi* is the state of *Chitta-Vritti-Nirodh* (Cessesion of the modifications of Mind).

Samprajnãta or *Sabija Samadhi* is outer part or the first stage of *Samadhi* and *Asamprajnãta* or *Nirbija Samadhi* is the inner *Samadhi* or the final stage of *Samadhi*.

12
Meditation: Revelation of Secrets of Nature

It is in the *Samprajnata Samadhi* that scientists make discoveries and inventions related to the Secrets of Nature (Prakriti). All the discoveries and inventions of the world are the results of deep meditation over a particular subject or problem. When Newton observed an apple falling on the ground, he retained this sight in his mind (concentration). He deeply contemplated on the phenomenon as to why it fell to the ground and why it did not fly into the sky. This deep thinking is Meditation (*Samadhi*). And the result was enlightenment. He perceived in this phenomenon of falling apple, the natural law of gravity in operation. Similarly, when Euclid, a great mathematician, was lying on his bed in a closed room looking vacantly at the walls around him, he went into deep state of meditation and gave to the world the plane geometry. One more example – James Watt sitting in his drawing room noticed the lid of a kettle on furnace jumping. He closely watched this phenomenon and contemplated upon it as to why the boiling water in the kettle was lifting the lid. He came to the conclusion that steam has force and, thus, the world got the steam engine and the railway system.

As indicated in the outset, Yoga is of two types – the Spiritual and the Secular. If one meditates upon Spiritual matters, one may advance spiritually; if one meditates upon material objects, one may make material progress and may even explore the secrets of Nature. The aforesaid instances are the examples of Secular Yoga.

13
Meditation: Source of Supernatural Powers

In the *Sabija Samadhi*, Yogi achieves some extraordinary powers. These powers are known as supernatural powers or psychic powers, e.g., ability to read one's mind, influence somebody's else mind; ability to communicate mentally with a person thousands of miles away (telepathy); ability to see things concealed at a distance, unknown places; levitation above the ground or even entering in another person's body. Given below are some examples:

(i) French Judge Louis Jacolliot on his visit to India saw a Yogi risen two feet above the ground and wondered: "For more than twenty minutes, tried to see how could he thus fly in the face and eyes of all known laws of gravity."

— 'Occult Science in India and Among the Ancients'.

(ii) In 1868, he (Daniel Home) was seen levitating out of a three-storey window; he floated back indoors through another window.

— Encyclopaedia of Mystical and Paranormal Experience.
— Rosemary Ellen Guiley

(iii) Apollo 14 Astronaut Edgar D. Mitchell conducted a telepathy experiment from space with four recipients on earth, 1,50,000 Miles below ...Mitchell concentrated on sequences of 25 random numbers. He completed 200 sequences .... two recipients had guessed 51 sequences correctly.

— Encyclopaedia of Mystical and Paranormal Experience.
— Rosemary Ellen Guiley

(iv) "I was in Hyderabad (Deccan) in India and I was told of a Brahmin there who could produce a number of things from where nobody knew. ..... twenty-five pairs of eyes stared at him. He said, "Now look, write down anything you desire." We all wrote down the names of fruits which never grew in that terrain. We gave him those bits of paper and there came under his blanket bushels of grapes, oranges and all sorts of fruits we demanded. ..... He ended his feet by producing a mass of roses, each flower was so perfect that it bore dew on its petals, as if it was freshly plucked from the garden.
It seemed impossible that it could be a sleight of hand."

— Vivekananda's Lectures

Quoted in 'Yogic Powers and God Realisation' by V.M. Bhatt

(v) Theosophist Colonel Alcott and Madame Vladovsky asked Swami Dayanand Saraswati whether it was a fact that Adi-Shankaracharya had entered the body of another person, Swami ji replied, "I do not know about its historicity, but entering the body of another person is possible by Yogic power. I can concentrate my Soul in the tip of my little finger and entering another person's body is only one step further. But I won't do it as it is prohibited for Yogis to indulge in such things."

— Srimad Dayanand Prakash (pg. 280) by Swami Satyananda

In the West, Psychics like Daniel Home, Robert Hudtchi, Rosa Kuleshova, Wolf Messing, Yuri Geller and many others who performed miraculous feats and exhibited supernatural powers, attracted the attention of philosophers and scientists. Editor of Nature magazine, David Davis commented, "In publishing the paper on Phenomenon of Yuri Geller, we are serving notice to the scientific community that there is something here worthy of their scrutiny."

(It needs to be clarified here that the supernatural powers possessed by the Western psychics are not the result of any Yoga *Sadhana*, but the faculties bestowed on them by birth. The Yogic term for this is JANMAJÃ SIDDHIS. The Siddhis acquired at birth are, in fact, the result of Yogic *Sadhana* done by them in the previous life. All the same, they all employed in their performances the potent weapon of concentration, EKAGRATA, which is a vital method of Yoga but the spiritual content of Yoga in these psychic powers is missing).

Deeply impressed by these psychic phenomena, Sigmund Freud stated, "I am now far from willing to repudiate these phenomena."

—Psychopathology of Everyday Life

"In the book 'Psychic Discoveries, Behind the Iron Curtain (page 52)', Sheila Ostrander and Lynn Schroeder stated "Sigmund Freud once remarked that if he had his life to live over again, he would have devoted it to psychic research".

These powers appear to be miracles, but actually they are performed through the agency of Nature which releases its powers to the elevated mind. Sage Patanjali terms it 'PRAKRITY ÃPÛRÃT' (23) (Filing up by Nature), Choa Kok Sui also expresses a similar opinion: "Miracles are fantastic events which utilise hidden laws of Nature that most people are not aware of. Miracles do not break the laws of Nature, they are actually based on them!." St. Augustine is also of the view, "Miracles are not contrary to Nature, but only contrary to what we know of Nature."

Though such divine powers can be achieved in Yoga, Sage Patanjali advises the Yoga practitioners not to use these because their exhibition generates egotism and, thereby, hampers spiritual progress in Yoga.

Thus Spake Plato

And thought is best when the mind is gathered into herself,
and none of these things trouble her –
neither sounds nor sights nor pain, nor any pleasure –
when she has as little as possible to do with the body
and has no bodily sense or feeling, but is aspiring after Being.

—Phaedo (Jowett's Translation)

14
Experiences in the Hour of Meditation (*Anubhuti*)

Samprajnata literally means to know everything in its true state as it is. *Samprajnata Samadhi* is like the dawn in which everything is visible except the Sun. That is why, in this state, the secrets of Nature are revealed and the secular practitioners make discoveries and inventions and attain supernatural powers.

Sabija or *Samprajnata Samadhi* is like the anti-chamber of the Sancto-Sanctum, *Nirbija* or *Asamprajnata Samadhi*. Greek Philosopher Plotinus has described this state thus. "Beginning with contemplation of corporal things in their multiplicity and harmony, it then retires upon itself and withdraws into the depth of its own being. .... But even there it does not find the Highest, the One." In this state of *Sampajnata Samadhi*, one has the foreknowledge of the impending Self-Realisation and God-Realisation.

God has been described in the Vedas as ÃDITYA-VARNAH, i.e., blazing like the Sun and in the Gita (11.12): DIVI SÛRYA SAHASRASYA BHAVED YUGAPAD UTTHITÃ (24), i.e., if the light of a thousand suns were to blaze forth at once in the sky, it will hardly match the blazing light of God. (Incidentally, dazzled by the light at the first experimental explosion of Atomic Bomb, Oppenheimer recited this Shaloka of Bhagwad Gita). It is, therefore, natural, that the practitioners of Yoga have some glimpse of it in the anti-chamber, the *Samprajnata Samadhi*, before they confront that blazing light in the *Asamprajnata Samadhi* where they realise God. Svetashvatar Upanishad (2.14) says that in the hour of meditation, Yoga practitioner experiences such faint glimpses of it:

NIHÃRA-DHÛMA-ARKA-ANILA-ANALÃNÃM
KHADYOTA-VIDYUT-SAFATIKA-SHASHÎNÃM
ETÃNI RÛPÃÑI PURAH-SARÃÑI
BRAMHAÑY ABHIVYKTI-KARÃÑI YOGE (25)

i.e., Fog, Smoke, the Sun, Wind, Fire, Glow-Warm, Lightening, a Crystal-ball, the Moon – these are the preliminary forms which produce the manifestation of Brahma, in Yoga.

We have said earlier that Yoga is not confined to Indians or Hindus. It has universal appeal and is meant for the whole humanity. The state of Samadhi has not only been experienced by the Indians, but also by many Western saints and saintly philosophers. The state of *Samadhi* could be of a few hours, even of a few weeks. The Indian *Yogis* are reticent to describe the state of *Samadhi* and their experiences gained in the hour of Meditation or Trance, the Ecstatic State. They simply say that it is as indescribable as is the taste of honey by a dumb person. They are reticent also because they do not want to exhibit their progress in Yoga *Sadhana* as it is prohibited, lest one should get trapped in egotism and fall off the path to *Moksha*. However, we do find expression of their experiences in deep meditation by Gurudev Rabindranath Tagore and some Western saintly philosophers as follows:

(i) "The *Yogis* could stay in a self-induced cataleptic state for weeks, whereas I could not stay in this condition for more than three days."

— Wolf Messing

(Psychic Discoveries Behind the Iron Curtain: Page 53).

(ii) "I am sure that there have come moments when my Soul has touched the infinite and has become intensely conscious of it through illumination of joy."

— Rabindranath Tagore

(iii) "I saw Eternity the other night,
Like a great ring of pure and endless light,
All Calm, as it was bright."

— Vaughan

(History of Western Philosophy by Bertrand Russell)

(iv) "The gate was opened that in one quarter of an hour, I saw and knew more than if I had been many years together at a University."

— Boehme

(v) "Standing on the bare ground, my head bathed by the blithe air, and uplifted into the infinite space – all mean egotism vanishes. I became a transparent eye-ball; I am nothing; I see all; the currents of the Universal Being circulated through me; I am part and particle of God."

— Emerson

(vi) "I experienced freedom, clarity and joy, I realised I was of time and eternity in equal measure. I was composed of physical matter and spiritual energy in equal measure."

— Robert Robin

(vii) "A kind of waking trance I have often had, quite from boyhood, when I have been all alone. This has generally come upon me through repeating my own name two or three times to myself silently, till all at once, out of the intensity of the consciousness of individuality, the individual itself seemed to dissolve and fade away into boundless being; and this was not a confused state, but the clearest of the clearest and the sweetest of the sweetest, the weirdest of the weirdest, utterly beyond words, where death was an almost laughable impossibility, the loss of personality (if so it were) seeming not extinction, but the only true life."

— Tennyson

Life of Tennyson, Vol. I, Page 320

(Quoted by Dr. S. Radhakrishnan in Indian Philosophy Vol. II, Page 858)

Thus Spake Thich Nhat Hanh

Meditating on the nature of creation and being, may be the best way to understand God.

15
Meditation: Way to Realisation of Self and God

It has been said repeatedly above that the real purpose of Yoga is the Union of Soul and God. That is why famous commentator of Yoga Darshana, Sage Vyasa has said: YOGAS-SAMADHI, i.e., Yoga is Samadhi – Meditation. Another commentator Yagyavalkya has said: SANYOGO YOGA ITY UKTO JIVĀTMA-PARAMĀTMANORITI (10), i.e., the Union of Soul and God is Yoga. German Philosopher Rudolf Steiner also expresses the same view: "Meditation is the way to knowing and beholding the eternal, indestructible, essential centre of our being."

Distinguishing *Nirbija Samadhi* from *Sabija Samadhi*, I.K. Taimni in his book 'The Science of Yoga' says: "In *Sabija Samadhi*, Seeker is really seeking Himself, but a veil, howsoever thin, still obscures his vision. In *Nirbija Samadhi*, He (Jivãtmã) attempts to tear off the last veil in order to obtain a completely unobstructed vision of Himself. This is what is meant by Self-Realisation."

Nirbija Samadhi is the final stage of Yoga when the *Vrittis*, the thought currents of mind come to a standstill. This is a state when the Seeds (*Sanskaras*) of *Karma* and *Avidya* are burnt out and mind has no basis to work upon. Dr. S. Radhakrishnan has described the *Chitta-Vritti-Nirodh*, thus, "The Yoga believes that the *Chitta* of man is like a millstone. If we put wheat under it, it grinds it into flour; if we put nothing under it, it grinds on until it grinds itself away" (Indian Philosophy Vol II page 362). In the *Nirbija Samadhi*, Mind or Prakriti loses its contact with Soul, thereby breaking the Cycle of Birth and Death. Now, Soul rests in itself and enjoys eternal bliss in the presence of God. Plato regards this ecstatic state "This Divine Madness" as the "Source of chiefest Blessings granted to man".

Greek philosopher Plotinus describes the final stage thus: "This (State of becoming one with God) is reached through contemplation of the primeval Being, the One. The last stage is reached when in the highest tension and concentration, beholding in silence and utter forgetfulness of all things, it is able, as it were, to lose itself. Then it may see God, the fountain of life, the source of being, the origin of all good, the root of the Soul. In that moment, it enjoys the highest indescribable bliss, it is, as it were, swallowed up of divinity, bathed in the light of Eternity."

How strikingly similar is this description of Plotinus to those of the Upanishads regarding Self-Realisation and God-Realisation!

To Sum Up

Yoga is a discipline which aims at one's physical, mental and spiritual development. It is beneficial for the individual as also for the society. It is essentially a spiritual discipline. The word 'Yoga' means union: Union of Self (Individual Soul) with God (the Supreme Being). In that state, the Individual Soul rests in eternal bliss. For this purpose, the Individual Soul has to make efforts. It is these requisite efforts which are known as Yoga Discipline. St. Angelus Silesius' words are very relevant in this context: "Man, if thou wishest to see God, there or here on earth, Thy heart must first become a pure mirror." Journey of Soul to God is a long and arduous one. Dag Hammer has rightly observed. "The longest Journey of any person is the journey inward." It is common knowledge that every journey starts with a first step. If one has the will and tenacity, the goal is not far to reach. The Gita (6.45) tells us that any little effort made in the Yoga practice, never goes waste and is carried forward to the next life and categorically assures us: ANEKA JANMA SANSIDHAS TATO YÃTI PRÃM GATIM (26) , i.e, after purifying oneself as per Yoga prescriptions and attaining perfection in the course of many lives, one reaches the highest destination – God.

This is, in short, the Philosophy of Yoga.

Section II

The Veda: God's Revelation
by Labi Bine Akhtab Bine Turfa

कवि का नाम
"लबी बिने अख्तब बिने तुर्फा"
अरब देश में हज़रत मुहम्मद से
२३०० तेईस सौ वर्ष पूर्व हुआ।

अया मुबारेकल अरज़ मुशैये नोहा मिनल हिन्दे।
व अरादकल्लाह मन्योनज्जेल जिकरतुन ॥१॥
वहलतज्जलीयतुन ऐनाने सहबी अरवे अतुन ज़िकरा।
वहाज़ेही योनज्जेल रसूल मिनल हिन्दतुन ॥२॥
यकूलूनल्लाहः या अहलल अरज़ आलमीन कुल्लहुम।
फत्तबेऊ ज़िकरतुल वेद हुक्कुन मालम योनज्जेलतुन ॥३॥
वहोवा आलमुस्साम वल युजुर मिनल्लाहे तनज़ीलन।
फऐनोमा या अख़ीयो मुत्तबेअन योबस्सीरीयोनजातुन ॥४॥
व इस्नैन हुमा रिक अतर नासेहीन का अ खुवातुन।
व अस्नात अला ऊदन व होवा मश ए रतुन ॥५॥
("सेअरुल्ओकूल" पृष्ठ [illegible])

(१) हे भारत की पुण्य भूमि! तू धन्य है क्योंकि ईश्वर ने अपने ज्ञान के लिये तुझको चुना।

(२) वह ईश्वर का ज्ञान प्रकाश जो चार प्रकाश स्तम्भों के सदृश सम्पूर्ण जगत् को प्रकाशित करता है, यह भारतवर्ष में ऋषियों द्वारा चार रूप में प्रकट हुआ।

(३) और परमात्मा समस्त संसार के मनुष्यों को आज्ञा देता है कि वेद जो मेरे ज्ञान है इनके अनुसार आचरण करो।

(४) वह ज्ञान के भण्डार साम और यजुर हैं जो ईश्वर ने प्रदान किये। इसलिये हे मेरे भाइयो इनको मानो क्योंकि ये हमें मोक्ष का मार्ग बताते हैं।

(५) और दो उनमें से रिक्, अतर (ऋग्, अथर्व) हैं जो हमको भ्रातृत्व की शिक्षा देते हैं, जो इनकी शरण में आ गया वह कभी अन्धकार को प्राप्त नहीं होता।
("सेअरुल्ओकूल" पृष्ठ [illegible])

The Veda: God's Revelation
Labi Bine Akhtab Bine Turfa

(Arab Poet of Antiquity : 2300 Years Before Prophet Mohammed)

AYÃ MUVÃREKAL ARAZ USHAIY NOHÃ MINAL HINDE.
VA ARÃDAKALLÃH : MAJYONAZZEL ZIKARATUN. (1)
VAHAL TAJLLÎYATUN AINANE SAHABI AKHATUN ZIKARÃ
VAHÃZEHÎ YONAZZELUL RASÛL MINAL HINDÛTUN. (2)
YAKÛ LÛNALLÃH : *YÃ AHALALA ARAZ ÃLMÎNA KULLAHUM.*
FATABEÛ ZIKARATUL VEDA HUKKUM MÃLAM YONAZELTVM. (3)
VAHOVÃ ÃLMUSSÃMA VALAYAJUR MINALLAHE TANAZÎLAN.
FA AINOMÃ YÃ AKHÎYO MUTTABEAN YOVASHSHERÎYO NAZÃTUN (4)
VA ISANAINA HUMA RIK ATAR NÃSEHÎNA KA AKHUVATUN.
VA ASANÃT ALÃUDANA BAHOVA MASHERTUN. (5)

(SE ARUL OKÛL Page 257)

1. O the sacred land of India! You are blessed
   because God has chosen you for His revelation.
2. God's illuminating revelation, that illumines the whole world like four lighthouses,
   manifested through the Sages in India in four forms (Vedas).
3. And God commands all human beings of the world to conduct themselves
   according to the Vedas which are My revelation.
4. Sama (Veda) and Yajur (Veda) are the repository of divine knowledge that God has bestowed.
   So my brethren! have faith in them as they show us the way to salvation.
5. And two of those are Rik (Rig Veda) and Attar (Atharva Veda) which teach us brotherhood.
   He who is enlightened by these will never beget darkness/ ignorance.

(SE ARUL OKÛL Page 257)

Mohenjo-daro Seal confirming Vedic Civilisation

DVÃ SUPARÑÃ SAYUJÃ SAKHÃYÃ
SAMÃNAM VRIKŠAM PARI ŠASVAJÃTE
TAYORANYAH PIPALAM SVÃDVATTI
ANSHNAN ANYO ABHI CHÃKSHÎTI. (27)

— Rig Veda (1.164.20)

Two friendly, beautiful birds are perched on the same tree. One of them enjoys the fruit of the tree and the other, without eating, watches keenly the accompanying one.

(The two Birds here are God and Soul and the Tree Nature.)

(The following Seal confirms that Mohenjo-daro Civilisation is Vedic Civilisation.)

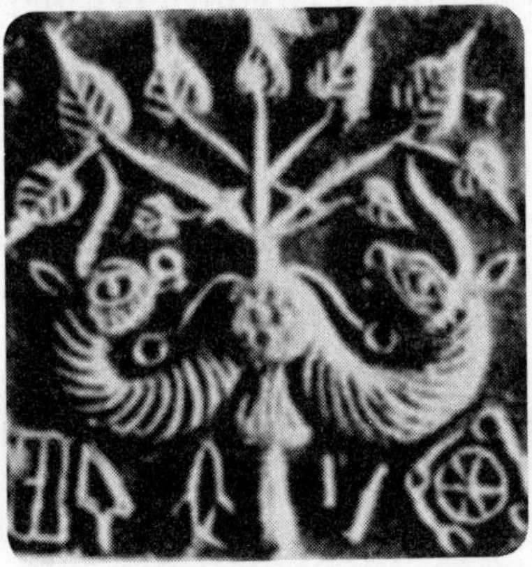

Photostat of Plate No CXII, Seal No. 387 from the excavations of Mohenjo-daro.

(From Mohenjo-daro and the Indus Civilisation edited by Sir John Marshall, Cambridge, 1931)

Vedic Nectar

MAHO ARÑAH SARASVATÎ
PRA CHETAYATI KETUNÃ
DHIYO VISHVÃ VI RÃJATI (28)

—Rig Veda 1.3.12

Vast is the Ocean of Sacred words
Which enlighten the intellects the world over
With divine vision.

16
The Fundamentals of Ancient Indian Philosophy

For the proper comprehension and practice of the philosophy of Yoga, it is essential to understand the fundamentals of the ancient Indian philosophy. These fundamentals are: Eternal existence of Three Entities, viz., *Ishvara* (God), *Jiva* (Individual Soul) and *Prakriti* (Nature) and operation of three Doctrines, viz., the Law of *Karma*, the Law of Reincarnation and the Law of Liberation. *Prakriti* (Nature) is *Sat* (Eternal) which is ever-existent but always changing its form. *Jiva* (Individual Soul) is *Sat-chit*, i.e., eternal and conscious. All flora and fauna are juxtapositions of *Prakriti* and *Jiva*. *Ishvara* (God) is *Sat-chit-Anand*, i.e., Eternal, Ever-conscious and Blissful. He is the Lord of all creation – animate and inanimate. *Prakrti* is *Ajna* (without Knowledge), *Jiva* is *Alpajna* (with limited Knowledge) and *Ishvara* is *Sarvajna* (Omniscient). The position of Soul is intermediary. It lacks bliss and is always craving for it. But owing to limited knowledge (ignorance), it mistakes sensory pleasure as bliss and runs into miseries. It makes certain endeavours to attain happiness which are known as *Karma* (actions). All individual Souls are responsible for their actions – good or bad and are rewarded or punished under the Law of Karma supervised by God. Soul acts through the agency of Mind which is a part of *Sukshma Sharira* (Astral Body). Every action leaves an imprint on the mind as does a foot leave an imprint on the sand it treads. These imprints form the nature of the mind and this nature further goads the mind to do more such actions. (Psychology also affirms that habits are formed by repeated actions). All these impressions called *Sanskaras* remain imbedded in the *Sukshma Sharira* (Astral Body) in the same manner as billions of data remain imbedded in a microchip of a computer. These impressions get activated at an opportune time. As reward or punishment for actions of one's whole life of an individual cannot be executed in one lifetime, Soul takes birth again and again, which is called the Law of Reincarnation. Soul carries in its astral body countless impressions of the deeds done in various births. The Soul takes birth in bodies of various species as per its deeds. The Cycle of Birth and Death continues until *Jiva* attains *Moksha* (Liberation) through realisation of God ie Brahma. In the state of *Moksha*, Soul rests in God in a blissful state. This state is known as being in Brahma-Loka.This period of *Moksha* is stated to be 36,000 cycles of creation and dissolution of the Universe. It then returns to the world and the Cycle of Birth and Death continues again. There will never be an end to the Cycle of Creation and Dissolution of the Universe.

Thus Spake Max Muller

"Vedas are the oldest text of the human race. And Agni Meele Purohitam is the first verse of Rig Veda. In the most primordial time, when the people did not know how even to cover their bodies and lived by hunting and housed in caves, Indians had attained high civilisation and they gave the world universal philosophies in the form of the Vedas".

17

Proofs of Existence of God

When Yoga is the union of Soul with God, it is incumbent on our part to first discuss whether God actually exists and what his traits, attributes and functions are. There are three types of people – Theists who believe in the existence of God, Atheists who do not believe in the existence of God and Agnostics who believe that God may or may not exist and that it cannot be conclusively proved either way. For the lay (who are not well versed in the religious or metaphysical matters), we put forward the following arguments:

(i) KÃRYA-KARTA-SAMBANDHA (Creation- Creator Relationship):

If there exists a thing, it must have been made by a maker. Seeing a good painting, we want to know who is its painter? Seeing a watch, we conclusively infer the existence of a watch-maker. Thus, seeing this universe, we can infer there must be a creator. Furthermore, cause and effect are interrelated. KÃRAÑÃBHÃVÃT KÃRYÃBHÃVAH (29), i.e., if there is no cause, there will be no effect. Our scriptures speak of three causes of the Universe – Material Cause (PRAKRITI – the Primordial Nature, the Holy Grail), Efficient Cause (God, who puts the holy grail in a purposeful order) and the Purpose (Bhogtã) – Enjoyer for whom this Universe has been made – the secondary Efficient Cause, otherwise why should God create the Universe. The following Mantra of the Rig Veda (10.72.2) will make this subject clear –

BRAHMAÑASPATIRETÃ SAM KARMÃRA IVÃDHAMAT
DEVÃNÃM PÛRVYE YUGE-ASATAH SADAJÃYATA (30)

i.e., the Lord of the Universe heated the elements like an ironsmith at the time of creation. And the invisible Nature (Prakriti) became visible. The Universe cannot be an act of Man because he appeared on the scene after the Creation, nor he has the knowledge and strength to do it. It must be some Omniscient, Omnipotent Entity to do it. In this context, words of Corpus Hermetica are worthy of attention: "The intellect makes itself visible in the act of thinking, God makes Himself visible in the act of Creating."

(ii) SRIŠTI-ÃYOJANA (Organisation in Creation)

Some argue that the elements of Nature can organise themselves into a Universe without the help of God, e.g., Fire emits light and heat without any assistance; Water can douse raging fire and a mixture of blue and yellow colours turns into green colour automatically. Undoubtedly, the elements of Nature have some distinct traits, but Nature itself is inanimate and has no knowledge even of itself. Blue and yellow colours lying in two tubes in a Laboratory cannot turn themselves into green except through the agency of a Lab Assistant.

The Vedanta Darshana (2.2.1-2) states: RACHANÃNUPAPATTE-SHCHA-NÃNUMÃNAM., PRAVRITTISHCHA. (31), i.e., Neither in experience nor by inference, creation has been seen to come into existence by itself, so Nature cannot be the efficient cause of the Universe. Secondly, for this is required, inclination/ desire to create, which is not there in Nature.

Renowned philosopher Flinch has had a penchant dig at the scientists who do not believe that God is the creator of the Universe. He says, "To believe that the atoms of Nature organised themselves into a fantastic universe is more unreasonable than to believe that the English language alphabets organised themselves into the great plays of Shakespeare without the help of the genius of Shakespeare. To believe that the atoms without the help of any principle or intelligent guidance created the universe comprising beautiful complex and beneficial objects is to cross the limit of blind faith that no greatest blind-believer of any religion has so far exhibited." Albert Einstein has categorically stated.

"Everyone who is seriously in the pursuit of science becomes convinced that a spirit is manifest in the laws of the Universe – a spirit vastly superior to man."

The first and the second arguments come under the Teleological Argument in the Western Philosophy.

(iii) SRIŠTI-DHRITI (Upholding of the Universe)

Science tells us the Earth is revolving around the Sun and is kept in its orbit by the law of gravitation. The Sun along with its planets and moons is revolving around our galaxy, Milky Way. Our galaxy containing billions of stars is travelling at a fantastic speed in the unlimited sky and so are the billions of galaxies along with their stars moving in the sky. Einstein also says all movement is relative. In relation to what/whom, they are moving? There must be some stationary power in relation to whom they are moving. And who holds the heavenly bodies together like pearls in a garland? The Atharva Veda (10.8.37) says:

YO VIDYÃT SÛTRAM VITATAM
YASMINOTÃH PRAJÃH IMÃH
SÛTRAM SÛTRASYA YO VIDYÃT
SA VIDYÃT BRAHMAÑAM MAHAT, (32)

i.e., one who knows this stretched string in which all heavenly objects are strung, and one who knows the string (power) behind the string, knows God, the Great. The same sentiment has been expressed in the Gita too: MAYI SARVAM IDAM PROTAM SÛTRE MAÑIGAÑÃ IVA, (33)

i.e., In Me all this is strung like pearls in a string.

(iv) SRIŠTI-VIDHÃN (Design in Creation)

There is Design, Order, Harmony, Purpose in the Universe which cannot come into existence by chance. The Rig Veda (10.190.1) says: RITAMCHA SATYAM CHA ABHÎDDHÃT TAPSO ADHYAJÃYAT (34), i.e., From the illuminating God flowed the Ritam (Eternal Cosmic Order) and Satyam (Essential Moral and Spiritual Laws). God's software of Rita and Satya governs the Universe incessantly without any error or exception. Albert Einstein also says: "I believe in God who reveals Himself in the orderly harmony of the Universe.

I believe that intelligence is manifested throughout in all Nature." Let us see, how?

a. In the physical world, Newton discovered the Law of Gravitation, but it existed right since the time of creation of the Universe, which holds the heavenly bodies in their orbits.

   Light travels at the speed of 1,86,281.7 miles per second, which has made communication so fast. Have the scientists put this limit of speed in light?

   Atom contains unfathomable energy which is now being tapped by the scientists, who stuffed that energy in the atom?

b. In the Vegetable Kingdom, we find a vast variety of fruits, vegetables, flowers, cereals, medicinal plants and what not. All have different shapes, sizes, nutrients, tastes and the like which are nourished by the same water, earth, sunlight, etc. Who designed all this?

c. In the animal kingdom, we have innumerable species of insects, birds, animals with mind-boggling variety. Glow-worm has a lifelong supply of electricity to glow. Bees have marvellous capacity to collect essence of flowers and convert it into honey for us. Dog has 10,000 times more powerful sense of smell than that of man that it now helps us to combat terrorism. Have we ever wondered at the unity in diversity in the entire animate world? Blood of all species is red and the milk of all milk-yielding animals is white. Medical science conducts tests of drugs on rats, frogs and monkeys, before introducing the same to humans. Not only that, all these species naturally transmit their own faculties in their respective progenies. Who has imbedded such faculties in them and devised this meticulous plan of transmission?

d. Homo sapiens is the crown of creation. All the parts of the body are unique and marvellous in themselves. The developed brain, the erect posture, faculty of language, the capacity to learn and transmit acquired knowledge from generation to generation – have enabled man to reach the Moon. Man boasts of his achievements. But was it all possible if He had willed human beings to crawl on the floor like other animals? We must recognise His existence and grace and say in admiration with Isaac Newton: "We are, therefore, to acknowledge one God-infinite, eternal, omnipresent, omnipotent, the creator of all things, most wise, most just, most good and most holy."

The above two arguments (iii and iv) come under Cosmological Argument in Western Philosophy.

(v) NYÃYÃ VIDHÃN (Dispensation of Justice)

Man is not only a rational animal, he is a justice-loving being too. All over the world, from the most advanced societies to the most illiterate, backward, tribal societies, there is a system of dispensing justice. There are courts or local bodies who punish the wily, crooked, thieves, murderers in all societies. There is no society which honours or rewards such persons. Whereas, the honest, philanthropists and virtuous persons are honoured and respected. Who has imbued sense of justice in Man? Yajurveda (19.77) says: ASHRADDHÃM ANRITE ADADHÃT SHRADDHÃM SATYE PRAJÃPATIH (35), i.e., God imbedded in man faith in Truth and aversion to Untruth.

Justice demands one should be rewarded for good deeds and punished for bad deeds. Judicial system depends on evidence. But judges are not omniscient. At times, miscarriage of justice happens because of false evidences. Justice demands there should be someone who is Omniscient, Omnipotent, Omnipresent. Sankhya Darshan (5.2) states: NA ÎSHVARA ADHIŠTHITE FALNIŠPATTIH KARMNÃ TATSIDHEH (36), i.e., Only under God's supervision-justice can be awarded, Deeds themselves can't bear fruits. Justice is seen to be done in His system, otherwise why one should be born crippled or healthy, rich or poor, ugly or beautiful?

Western philosopher Emmanuel Kant puts forth moral argument about the existence of God thus, "A justly proportioned distribution of rewards and punishment can only be expected from an infinite power, wisdom and goodness which rules the moral world even as it has created the natural world... The atheist is blind to the intimate connection which exists between the highest good and the Idea of Reason; he does not see that God, Freedom and Immorality (of Soul) are the indispensable conditions of the realisation of this ideal."

(vi) All Religions have Faith in God

All the religions of the world believe in the existence of God and instruct their followers to pray and sing praises of Him. The religious texts of different religions speak of their masters having realised God. This in itself is a sound proof of existence of God.

(vii) Whole Humanity Believes in God

Leaving aside a few self-proclaimed atheists, nearly the whole of humanity believes in the existence of God. From the great philosophers like Plato, Kant to the illiterate tribal men, all believe in God. In Mahatma Gandhi's words, "Each one prays to God, according to his own light."

"Never has man lived without God; if you remove one, he will create another."

— Tolstoy

"If there is no God, let us create one."

— Emerson

"I have been driven many times to my knees by the overwhelming conviction that I have nowhere else to go."

— Abraham Lincoln

When Apollo 13 suffered leakage of oxygen, the great scientists of NASA were ringing bells in churches for the astronauts' safe return. People all over the world were praying in their own way for their safe return. Is this fact not a convincing proof of mankind's belief in God? Spontaneous utterances 'O My God!', 'Ya Allah!', 'Hey Prabhu!' from the depth of men's heart all over the world are indeed a potent proof of existence of God.

(viii) Voice of Conscience

Voice of one's Conscience is yet another potent proof of the existence of God. When a man does something ethically wrong, he feels fear and self-pity, but when a man does something good, he feels enthused and elated. Furthermore, one has the tendency to do good deeds in public and bad deeds when nobody is seeing him, being oblivious of the fact that an Invisible Eye is seeing all he does.

"The entity which experiences these feelings is Soul and the entity which evokes these feelings is God."

— Swami Dayanand Saraswati

"When I do good, I feel good. When I do bad, I feel bad. That is my religion."

— Abraham Lincoln

"God talks incessantly. But as it turns out, Mankind is deaf."

— Don Williams Jr.

"A Touchstone God has placed in every heart it separates, with surety, False from True."

— Sufi Poet

(ix) Source of the Initial Knowledge (Veda)

It is well known that Man gets knowledge through parents, teachers and society. By himself he cannot attain knowledge. We got knowledge from our teachers; they from their teachers and so on ad absurdum. Who gave the initial knowledge to the first human beings on earth? *Yoga Darshana* (1.26) replies – PÛRVEŠÃMAPI GURUH KÃLENA AN-AVACHHEDÃT (37), i.e., He is the teacher of all previous teachers, being unaffected by Time. The *Vedanta Darshana* (1.3) also affirms: SHÃSTRA-YONITVÃT (38), i.e., God's existence is proved by being the source of Veda, initial knowledge. The following statements of renowned philosophers also point to the same conclusion:

"If there is a God who has created Heaven and Earth, it will be unjust on His part, if he deprives millions of His sons born before Moses, of his divine knowledge. Reason and Comparative study of religions declare that God gives His divine knowledge from his (Man's) first appearance on Earth."

— F. Max Muller (Science and Religion)

"The Vedas, I feel convinced, will occupy scholars for centuries to come, and we take and maintain for ever its position as the most ancient of books in the library of mankind."

— F. Max Muller (India : What Can It Teach Us?)

"After the latest researches into the history and chronology of books of the Old Testament, we can safely now call the Rig Veda as the oldest book, not only of the Aryan humanity, but of the whole world... We are justified, therefore, in concluding that the higher and purer conceptions of the Vedic Aryans were the results of a primitive Divine Revelation."

— Rev Morris Philip (The Teaching of the Vedas)

The following words of an Arab Poet 2,300 years before Prophet Mohammed, when there was no Islam, no Christianity, no Judaism, no Zoroastrianism, categorically declare Vedas as the revelation of God:

"O the sacred Land of India! You are blessed because God has chosen you for his revelation. God commands all human beings of the world to conduct themselves according to the Vedas which are My revelation."

— Labi Bine Akhtab Bine Turfa (Se-arul Okool, page 157)

(x) Anubhûti Pramãña (Self- Realisation Argument)

Now the question arises if God exists, why can't we see him? The answer is: Do we see hunger? No, we can only experience it. Similarly, God cannot be seen, He can only be experienced. Who can experience him? Not the eyes, not the physical senses. God being non-material entity can only be seen/experienced by a non-material entity viz., Soul. Shvetashvatar Upanishad (2.15) says:

YADÃ ÃTMATATTVENA TU BRAHMATATTVAM
DÎPOPAMENEHA YUKTAH PRAPASHYET
AJAM DHRUVAM SARVA-TATTVAIR VISHUDDHAM
JNYÃTVÃ DEVAM MUCHYATE SARVA-PÃSHAIH, (39)

i.e., When a Yogi by means of the real nature of his self, sees, as if by a lamp here, the real nature of Brahma, by knowing God, who is unborn, eternal, free from all nature (material trapping), he is released from all fetters.

St. Thomas Aquinas has also expressed the same sentiment thus: "In order to see God, there is needed some likeness of God on the part of the visual power, whereby the intellect becomes capable of seeing God."

— Summa Theologica

The above experience of God relates to the Yogis and the highly spiritually evolved Souls. The question arises how can an ordinary person experience/see God? The answer to this question has been exquisitely given by thinker Pearl Bailey, "People see God everyday, they just don't recognise Him." Now we give below some facts which prove that the above statement is absolutely true.

Man lives in three states – wakeful state, dream state and dreamless state (*Sušupati*) and surprisingly experiences God daily in all these states, but unfortunately is unaware of his experience of God.

a. In wakeful state, at every step, man experiences God in the form of voice of his conscience which prohibits him from doing anything sinful.
b. In dream state, mind, along with all senses, resides in the astral body (*Sukšma Sharira*) and, at times, sees dreams imparting enlightening secrets, e.g., Neil Bohr became aware of atom's structure in a dream. Such secrets/ inspirational ideas are revealed by God. *Yoga Darshana* (1.38) advises SVAPNA NIDRÃ JNÃNÃLAMBANAM VÃ (40), i.e., by pondering over the knowledge received in dream-state or dreamless state, one can make progress in Yoga.
c. In dreamless sleep called *Sušupti*, mind goes to sleep and rests in KÃRANA SHRIRA (Causal Body). Soul rests in its *Ãnandamaya Kosha* (Blissful Sheath) and feels extremely peaceful and blissful. *Sankhya Darshana* (5.116) says:SAMÃDHI-SUŠUPATI-MOKŠEŠU BRAHMARÛPTÃ (41), i.e., in *Samadhi*, *Sušupti* and *Moksha*, Soul attains likehood to God.

To sum up, God exists and one experiences Him. Having full faith in Him, aspirant of Yoga will make tremendous progress in this journey to Self-Realisation.

18
Nature, Attributes and Functions of God

Rig Veda says 'EKAM SAT VIPRÃH BAHUDHÃ VADANTI (42), i.e., God is one, the wise call Him by many names. His personal name is AUM, which means the Protector. AVATI RAKŠTI ITI AUM (43), i.e., one who saves is AUM. Yoga *Darshana* and other scriptures advise aspirants to chant this name, meditating on its meaning. All sages and saints are said to have chanted AUM and meditated on Him. God has many attributes and functions. Accordingly, He has many names which, in fact, represent His faculties, attributes and functions. Swami Dayanand Saraswati, in his magnum opus Satyarth Prakash explains 100 names of God along with their meanings, e.g., He is Brahma, being supreme; Vishnu, being omnipresent; Shiva, being benevolent; Svayambhu, being Self-born – has no father or mother; Janita, being progenitor of everything; Vidhata, being organiser of everything; Ishvara, being Ruler of the Universe; Indra, being source of wealth; Parmatama, being the Supreme Being; Prana, being the source of all energy; Rudra, being one who makes the evil doers weep; Shukra, being extremely pure; Agni, being the source of light and knowledge; Vayu, being all mighty; Varuna, being dispenser of Justice; Hiranyagarbha, being the womb of all heavenly bodies; Kala, being the counter of everything; Yama, being as it were, the ledger keeper of all actions of all beings. Jataveda, being revealer of the Veda for guidance of humanity; Jagadamba, being the mother of the Universe. And finally, EKA EVA NAMASYAH (44), i.e., Only One (as stated above) is worthy of being adorned and worshipped.

All these names are the names/faculties of God, but by the passage of time, they were regarded as different deities and, thereby, incurring the charge of Polytheism. This has been resolutely refuted by Swami Dayanand in the first chapter of Satyarth Prakash as also by Prof. F. Max Muller thus: "They were all meant to express the Beyond, the Invisible, the Infinite within the Finite, the Supernatural above the Natural, the Divine, Omnipresent and Omnipotent."

— India: What Can It Teach Us?

That is what the Atharva Veda (13.4.21) says: SARVE ASMIN DEVÃH EK VRITTO BHAVANTI (45), i.e., All the Devas (forces) become One, reflect the One.

God's all actions are for the benefit of His children. God is not bound by the fruits of His actions. Yoga *Darshana* (I. 24) says: KLESHA KARMA VIPÃKÃSHAIR-APARÃMRIŠTAH PURUŠA VISHEŠA ÎSHVARAH (46), i.e., one who is unaffected by sufferings, fruit of action, desire to enjoy fruit is the peculiar person called God.

In short, God's functions (*Karma*) are five:

a) To create the Universe, being *Srišti-Kartã*
b) To uphold, sustain and maintain the Universe, being *Srišti-Dhartã*.
c) To dissolve the Universe after expiry of its lifespan, being Srišti-Sanhartã.
d) To dispense justice to all beings according to their actions, being *Karma Adhyaksha*.
e) To impart divine knowledge (*Veda*) at the time of creation, for the guidance of humanity, being *Jãtaveda*.

Although God's attributes are innumerable, for purposes of practical knowledge, a few – Omniscient, Omnipotent, Omnipresent, Immortal, Merciful, Kind, Benevolent and Just – can cater for all the above activities of God. All religions of the world express the same sentiments about God. Different names in different religions, more or less, express the same meaning, e.g., the words God in Christianity, Jahova in Judism, Ahur Masda in Zoroastrianism, Allah or Khuda in Islam, Rab, Omkar or Vaheguru in Sikhism. In this context, the words of Shakespeare are most relevant: "Rose by any other name will smell as sweet."

Now the question arises how God operates in this vast Universe and rules over the innumerable Souls in it? Answer to this question can be seen partly in the arguments under the Subsection 'Proofs of Existence of God'. All the same, some more light on this question will be in order.

Yajur Veda (40.8) describes the personality of God thus:

SA PARYAGÃT SHUKRAM AKÃYAM
AVRAÑAM ASNÃVIRAM SHUDDHAM APÃPVIDDHAM
KAVIR MANÎŠÎ PARIBHÛH SVAYAMBHÛR
YÃTHÃTATHYATO ARTHÃN VYADADHÃT
SHÃSHVATÎBHYAH SAMÃBHYAH (47)

i.e., He is all-pervading, extremely powerful, without body, without veins and arteries, extremely pure, unaffected by any sin, Omniscient, aware of workings of the minds of all, Omnipresent, Self-born (has no father or mother), for all His subjects the world over, imparted the right knowledge (Vedas) for the guidance.

Shvetãshvatar Upanishad (3.19) gives us some idea how He functions:

APÃÑI-PÃDO JAVANO GRAHÎTÃ
PASHYATI ACHAKŠU SA SHRIÑOTY-AKARÑAH
SA VETTI VEDYAM NA CHA TASYA ASTI VETTA
TAM ÃHUR AGRYAM PURUŠAM MAHÃNTAM. (48)

i.e., He grasps without hands; moves fast without feet; sees without eyes; and He listens without ears. He knows whatever is knowable, but there is no one who knows Him; Him they call Primeval Supreme Person.

All the same, even if He has no hands or feet or eyes or ears, yet He works so meticulously as if He had thousands of heads, eyes, ears and feet all functioning in unison. Yajur Veda (31.1) says

SAHASRASHÎRŠÃ PURUŠAH
SAHASRÃKŠAH SAHASRAPÃT
SA BHÛMIM SARVATA SPRITVÃ
ATYATIŠTHAD DASHÃNGULAM (49),

i.e., The Supreme Being has, as it were, thousands of heads, thousands of eyes and thousands of feet. He, having pervaded the whole Universe, transcends and resides in the hearts of everyone. (Word '*Dashãngul*' stands for the animate being with five Pranas, mind, intellect, consciousness and will power).

To sum up, God works on His own, because of His Omniscience, Omnipotence and Omnipresence. He works through His software of *Rita* and *Satya* – Eternal Cosmic Laws and Eternal Moral and Spiritual Laws. And yet NA TASYA PRATIMÃSTI YASYA NÃMA MAHADYASHAH (50) (Yajur Veda 32.3), i.e., whose name evokes so much of glory and fame, has no image, is invisible. He is only to be felt and adored in the hearts.

Thus Spake Buddha on Brahma

"Brahma am I, Great Brahma, the Supreme.
The Unsurpassed, Perceiver of All Things,
Controller, Maker, Fashioner, Lord of All
Chief, Victor, Ruler, Father of All Beings
That ever has been, are and are to be!"

—Kevatta-Sutta, Dîgha Nîkâya

(The Bible of Bibles Page 115, by Dr. F.L. Riley)

Thus Spake Ãdi Shankrâcharya on God

O God! Pardon me three things :
I have in contemplation clothed in form Thyself without form;
I have in praise described Thee who transcends all qualities;
And in visiting shrines, I have ignored Thy omnipresence.

19
Nature and Activities of Soul (JIVA)

In the Vedas and the Upanishads, Soul has many names, which duly reflect its nature and activities. It is called JIVA (Living Being) ATMAN (Being), PURUŠA (Living in a body), KARTÃ (Doer), BHOGTÃ (Enjoyer of fruits of action), DRASTÃ (Seer), CHITI (Conscious), PRÃNÎ (Breather), AJA (Unborn), AJAR (Does not get old), AMAR (Immortal), TAT (That), SAT (Eternal), etc. (Word 'ÃTMÃ' is masculine in Sanskrit and feminine in Hindi).

Soul is the source of life. When Soul enters a body, it becomes live or animate; when it leaves it, it becomes a dead body. Presence of Soul in a body generates activity as, for example, in an amoeba. Science's dictum is: 'Activity is the manifestation of life'. Aristotle has justly defined Soul thus: "The Soul is that thing that determines, by its presence or absence, what is alive and what is not." Soul distinguishes itself from matter by its consciousness. That is why Adi Shankaracharya has affirmed: "We can doubt or deny any object, but we cannot deny one's own being, for in the very act of doubting or denying, we affirm our existence." Descartes has also said, "Cogito Ergo Sum", i.e., "I think, therefore, I am." *Nyaya Darshana* and Vaishešik Darshana enumerate the following traits of Soul, i.e., inhalation and exhalation, affection and disdain, pain and pleasure, efforts and knowledge.

Soul is said to have three activities:

Gyãtritva (To know), *Kritritva* (To act) and *Bhogtritva* (To enjoy). Soul being *Alpagya*, i.e., with limited knowledge has the tendency to know more and more. As per the level of his knowledge, he acts. As he acts, so does he reap the fruits of his action in the form of pleasure and pain. Soul lives in three states – *Sharîrãvasthã,* i.e., in body form, *Pretyãvasthã,* i.e., in body-less state when it leaves a body on death and travels to acquire another body; it is more or less an unconscious state when he feels no pleasure or pain; this is also the state during the *Pralaya* –dissolution of the Universe. Third state is *Mokshãvasthã,* i.e., state of liberation or salvation. In this state, he is all-blissful and enjoys the company of God.

Soul acquires three bodies – *Sthûl Sharira,* i.e., gross, physical body, which we all possess now, *Sukshma Sharira,* i.e., Astral Body. It is that body with which he travels to an unknown destination after death. All the impressions (*Sanskaras*) of various lives remain imprinted in this body and those impressions spring up to goad him to act in accordance with the experiences of previous lives. The third is *Kãrana Sharira,* i.e., Causal Body. This is that body where the mind goes to sleep and rests in it in *Sušupti,* dreamless state. Causal body is made of Nature (*Prakriti*) in its primordial state. *Karana Sharira,* causal body is common to all. The following statement of thinker Bill Bryson gives us the feel what causal body is: "Atoms are fantastically durable. Because they are so long-lived, atoms really get around. Every atom you possess has almost certainly passed through several stars and been part of millions of organisations on its way to becoming you. We are each atomically so numerous and so vigorously recycled at death that a significant number of atoms – up to a billion for each of us; it has been suggested – probably once belonged to Shakespeare. A billion more each came from Buddha and Chenghis Khan and Beethoven, and any other historical figure you care to name… So, we are all reincarnations – though short-lived ones. When we die, our atoms will disassemble and move off to find new uses elsewhere – as part of a leaf or human being or drop of dew. Atoms themselves, however, go on practically forever."

— A Short History of Everything

Souls are innumerable but are identical. *Shatpath Brãhmana* says, NA JYEŠTHÃSAH NA KANIŠTHÃSAH ETE. (51), i.e., they are neither big nor small; neither superior nor inferior. Soul of an elephant is not bigger than the Soul of an ant; nor the Soul of a man is superior to the Soul of an ass. Chhãndogya Upanishad (6.9.3-4) says: This tiger, this lion, this wolf, this insect, this fly – all have an *Atman*

(Soul), telling the disciple TAT TVAM ASI (52), i.e., Thou art that, meaning thereby, your Soul is identical with theirs.

If all are identical, then why is the difference? That is because of *Karmas*, good or bad deeds. Soul acquires various forms of life according to his deeds in innumerable lives. Furthermore, Soul has no gender – male, female or neutral. Chhandogya Upanishad (6.9.3) says TVAM STRÎ TVAM PUMÃNASI (53), i.e., you are a woman, you are a man. (In modern days, change of sex by individuals affirms this). A male person may be born a female or vice versa in next life. Soul acquires gender according to one's deeds in various lives.

While in the Vedas, the Upanishads, the Gita, or any other scripture, there is no mention of the number of life-forms in which Soul manifests itself; in the Garura Purana, there is a mention of 84 lakh *Yonis*, i.e., 8.4 million life-forms. It is surprising that science also believes that there are 8-10 million species of flora and fauna. Soul is eternal and it eternally keeps on appearing in one life-form or the other and gains experiences in these life-forms. Experiences gained and the desire to relive those experiences is called *Vasana*. Yoga *Darshana* (4.10) says TÃSÃM ANÃDITVAM CHÃSHÎŠO NITYATVÃT (54), i.e., the *Vasana* has no beginning and the desire to live being eternal. Relevant *Vasanas* keep on appearing on Soul's entering the concerned life-forms. Otherwise, how is it that a newborn bird starts flying shortly after birth and a newborn child sucks milk from the mother's breast? This proves that all Souls have manifested themselves in all forms of life at one time or the other.

The Brihadaranyaka Upanishad (4.4.3) states that at the time of death, Soul is aware of which life-form it is going to get. It says just as a caterpillar before leaving the leaf it is perched on, gets hold of another leaf. Similarly, Soul gets attracted towards the new life-form before leaving the present body (death). At the time of death, man visualises in a kaleidoscopic way his whole life. As it were, God is reading out the judgement as does a judge read out the charges against the culprit before passing the judgement. Rudolf Steiner also expresses the idea of the preview of the forthcoming life thus: "Before the spiritual seed of the physical body descends to the parents who have been chosen to receive it, the Soul is granted a vision of life to come."

— (The Case for Reincarnation Page 12.3 – Joe Fisher).

Furthermore, The Tibetan Book of the Dead states: "When birth as a beast is imminent, the soul 'will see, as if through a mist, rock-caves and holes in the ground and straw huts'."

Zoroastrian Prayer

May Ahurâ give us the truth of Brahm
May He unite us with that Absolute,
When we have undergone successfully
The disciplines whereby the Vice in us
Is overthrown by Virtue, which make man
Divinely meritorious, and which bring
Salvation unto man and gods alike.

—*Gâthâ 46.17*

20
Is Time of Death Pre-determined?

Lastly, a question is often asked whether the mode and time of death is pre-determined. With some people, it is an article of faith that time and mode of death is predetermined. But if we critically analyse this, we may come to the other conclusion. First, all scriptures, health manuals advise that living a balanced life will increase the life span. Second, all the scriptures contain prayers for long life; if the life span cannot be extended, these prayers will become futile. Third, if time and mode of death are pre-determined, then a murderer extinguishing his victim's life, is only executing the will of God, why should he be punished? For example, if Prime Minister Indira Gandhi was destined to die on that fateful day in the manner she did, why were her assassins awarded death sentence? They only executed the will of God. Thus, the belief that time and mode of one's death is pre-determined makes the judicial system fall flat. This belief is against all the canons of common sense and against any society's norms.

Dr. Deepak Chopra's Views on Life Span

Our lifespan based on the conditioning and tendencies we come in with is not necessarily determinant in exactly how long we live. It is just a working set of programmed probabilities. The choices we make influence our lifespan. Depending on the particular Karmas associated with the life plan, the decisions we make can impact the length and the quality of life we live.

21
Where is the Soul Located in the Body?

Different cultures have different notions about where the Soul dwells in the body. For example, in many tribal cultures, blood has been associated with Soul. The Greek historian Herodotus records that the Scythians ritually drank the blood of their victims to absorb their courage and virtue. Similarly, Head also has a long association with Soul. That is why, to propitiate the gods, head of an animal became an essential part of animal sacrifice. For some cultures, the Soul dwelt not in blood or head, but in breath. Marquesans and New Caledonians used to hold the mouth and nose of dying people closed, in an effort to keep them alive, by keeping them ensouled. Modern scientists, who believe in the existence of Soul, also believe that it dwells in the brain, because when the brain is dead, Man is virtually dead.

But the ancient Indian scriptures tell us that the Soul dwells in the pit below the diaphragm. The Bhagvad Gita (18.61) says: ÎSHVARAH SARVA BHÛTÃNÃM HRID-DESHE ARJUN TIŠTHTI (55), i.e., O Arjun! God dwells in the HRID-DESH of every being. In the *Shankhayan Aranyak*, it is stated ÃTMANI BRAHMA (56), i.e., God resides in the Soul. So, by extension, Soul also resides in the Hrid-desh, the seat of Brahma. It is clarified here that Hrid-desh is not heart as heart-transplants confirm this. Swami Dayanand Saraswati has stated that Soul resides in the pit of the diaphragm, which is quite close to the heart but not the heart itself. It is known as *Brahmapuri* because *Brahma* (God) resides there. It is also known as *Indrapuri* because *Indra* (Soul) resides there. It is also known as *Tripuri* because God, Soul and Nature all three reside there. It is also known as *Guha* (cave/secret place) and *Anahat Chakra*.

Surprisingly, irrespective of any country or culture one belongs to, all human beings the world over when boastfully refer to 'I', e.g., I did it; I can do it, invariably and inadvertently, point their fingers to the pit below the diaphragm. Does this not confirm the truth, the Indian scriptures have revealed, that Soul resides in the pit below the diaphragm?

Pearls of Wisdom

Study the past,
If you would divine the future

—Confucius

Life is like a game of chess,
which changes with every move.

—Chinese Proverb

Goodness is the only investment that never fails.

—Henry Thoreau

22

Relationship between God and Soul

Relationship between God and Souls is unique. No errant Soul can run away from the Kingdom of God. Nor God, despite being Omnipotent, can expel an errant Soul from His Kingdom. Atharva Veda (10.8.32) says: ANTI SANTAM NA JAHÃTY ANTI SANTAM NA PASHYATI (57), i.e., Supreme Lord is too near to be abandoned and too close to be witnessed. Their relationship is three-fold – One, PITÃ-PUTRA SAMBANDHA, i.e., Father-Son Relationship; Two, RÃJÃ-PRAJÃ SAMBANDHA, i.e., King-Subject Relationship; Three, UPÃSYA-UPÃSAKA SAMBANDHA, i.e., Lord-Devotee Relationship. All religions believe that we are children of God. God, the kind Father, makes arrangement for feeding the newly born child by welling-up milk in his mother's breast at his birth. Before animals and humans appeared on earth, He ensured for them vegetables, fruits, cereals and the like. We, the children, seek our father's guidance in difficult situations. The great Father, sitting in our consciences, guides us what is right and what is wrong.

However, when a child errs, Father or Mother gives him a slap in his own interest. Similarly, kind Father, God, punishes us for our good. However, when an incorrigible son deliberately and persistently violates the laws of the Father, He assumes the role of a King and treats His son as a subject. His Law of *Karma* then comes into action in full force. Even in that, God is merciful for, as the Bible says "God brings men into deep waters, not to drown them, but to cleanse them."

Sooner or later, all Souls have to go to the lap of their Father. For this, the door open is of Lord-Devotee relationship. Dong Horton reminds us, "We are all serving a life sentence and good behaviour is our only hope for a pardon." When an errant Soul sincerely realises the futility and folly of his sinful pursuits, he returns to the virtuous life; he bows to God for forgiveness; follows the Yogic precepts like *Ishvara Pranidhan* (Devotion to God) and adopts service of humanity as service of God.

Now the chastened devotee prays to God –

ASTOMÃ SAD GAMAYA,
TAMSO MÃ JYOTIR GAMAYA,
MRITYOR MÃ AMRITAM GAMAYA (5),
i.e., O God!
Lead me from untruthful life to truthful life,
Lead me from darkness to light,
Lead me from mortality to immortality.

The Holy Bible (John 17.5) has a similar prayer:

"And now, O Father, Glorify thou me with Thine own self, with the glory which I had with thee before the world was."

There is no other way, all humanity seeks his shelter. A Sufi poet has said:

"Muslims, Christians or Jews or good or bad
All turn their eyes to the eternal one."

And God listens to the prayers of the chastened child and he returns to Him – The *Param Dham*. This is what is meant by Paradise Regained.

Soul's relationship with God as also its relationship with Nature (*Prakriti*) are well illustrated in the Parable of Adam and Eve in the Garden of Eden. Adam and Eve are the Souls and the Garden of Eden is the Paradise or the blissful presence of God where they are residing. Apple is the symbol of *Prakriti* – Nature's bounty which attracts the Souls for its enjoyment. *Satan* is the *Trishna* (Desire or Craving for enjoyment). When Adam and Eve fall prey to *Satan* (*Trishna*) and taste the so-called forbidden fruit – Nature's attraction, they forego the right to live in the presence of God, Paradise. And they come to this world and undergo sufferings. But the situation is not irretrievable. There is the Son of God (Conscience) to help them regain Paradise. One has to follow the dictates of one's conscience as also to follow the teachings of the Enlightened Souls, to regain Paradise. Son of God, Christ's Sermon on the Mount (10 Commandments) is exactly the *Yama* and *Niyama* of Yoga *Darshana*. Following the Yogic path of

Moral Discipline and Meditation on the Supreme Being is the only way to get back to Paradise: TAMEVA VIDITVÃ ATIMRITYUM ETI NÃ ANYAH PANTHÃ VIDYATE AYNÃYA (58) (Yajur Veda 31.18), i.e., by knowing Him alone, One can overcome Death, there is no other way to reach the Original Home. This is Paradise Regained.

Thus Spake a Sufi Poet

CHÎST DUNIYÃ ?
AZ KHUDÃ GÃFIL SHUDAN
NA Î KE MÃSH O NUKRAH
O FARZAND O ZAN
(The 'world' is but forgetfulness of God.
It is not spouse and child, silver or gold.)
(Essential Unity of All Religions page 24 : Bhagwan Das)

23
God and Souls – Entirely Different Entities

God is one and Souls are many. *Sankhya Darshana* (1.1.09.114) says: JANMÃDI VYAVASTHÃTAH PURUŠÃ BAHUTVAM (59), i.e., owing to differences in the species as also differences at birth, the Souls are many, e.g., some are born as humans, some as animals and some as insects and furthermore, some are born healthy, some crippled; some ugly and some beautiful; some genius and some imbeciles. They all cannot be one but different entities, so Souls are many.

They all are not only different from each other, they are entirely different from God. God is Omniscient, Souls have limited knowledge; God is Omnipresent, Souls are present at specific places; God is Omnipotent, Souls have limited strength and capacity. God is all bliss, Souls suffering from death, disease and hunger are always craving for bliss.

Pointing out the differences between God and Souls, Yoga *Darshana* (1.24) says: KALESH KARMA VIPÃKÃSHAIR APARÃMRIŠTAH PURUŠA-VISHEŠA ÎSHVARAH (46), i.e., Ishvara is a Distinct Person who is untouched by the afflictions of life, actions, and the results and impressions produced by these actions. (In Vedas and Upanishads, God and Soul are both called *Puruša*; hence, God here has been referred to as a Distinct Person).

There is a school of thought called ADVAITAVÃDA (Non-Dualism). They believe that there is only One Entity called *Brahma* (God) which under the influence of *Maya/Avidya* takes the form of many JIVAS (Souls). Now the question arises how Omniscient

God gets affected by *Avidya*/Ignorance and forgets His own true identity? How God who is all-bliss (*Ãnanda-Svarûp*) and immutable (NIRVIKÃRA) gets changed and becomes miserable. If it is said in defence that it is all His 'play' (LEELÃ), then God appears to be an innocent, ignorant child who cuts his finger while playing with a knife. Furthermore, *Maya* appears to be a different Entity than God which contradicts the ADVAITA's postulate, viz., Non-Dualism. Not only that, *Maya* appears to be more powerful than the Omnipotent God, which converts the Omniscient into an *Alpagya Jiva* (Soul with limited knowledge). Still further, if all *Jivas* are *Brahma*, then the distinction between the murderer and the murdered gets obliterated, thereby making the judicial system, the world over, irrelevant. And if *Jiva* (Soul) is no other than *Brahma* (God), then the relationship between *Bhagt* and *Bhagwan* (Lord and the Devotee) disappears, making prayers in all the Holy Books of the world futile.

In support of this postulate that God and Souls are one, some quote the Gita's *shloka* (15.7) MAMAIVÃNSHO JÎVALOKE JÎVABHÛTAH SANÃTANAH (60), i.e., a fragment (or fraction) of My own Self, having become a living Soul, eternal, moves in the world of life. While explaining the term 'MAMAIVANSHA', Dr. S. Radhakrishnan says, "This does not mean that the Supreme is capable of division or partition into fragments ... (it means) the reality of individual Soul is Divine... When he rises above his limitations, he is not dissolved in the Superpersonal Absolute but lives in the supreme." The Gita also states: NIVASIŠYASI MAYI EVA (61), i.e., You will reside in Me. It means Soul is different from God. Adi Shankaracharya himself interprets it as ANSHA IVÃNSHO NA HI NIRAVAYAVASYA MUKHYO ANSHAH SAMBHAVATI (62), i.e., the meaning of ansha is 'like an ANSHA', not that it is main Ansha of the immutable, which is not possible. The Gita's term 'MAMAIVANSHA' only means God-like. It is not like a particle of fire which has all the qualities of fire. Soul is divine, AMRITASYA PUTRÃH (4) (Son of the Immortal) not God Divine Himself.

To sum up, the *Advaita's* assertion JIVOBRAHMETI NETRAH (63), i.e., *Jiva* (Soul), verily, is *Brahma*, no other – is not logical, nor it is in accordance with the tenets of Vedas. Rig Veda (1.164.20) categorically declares:

DVÃ SUPARNÃ SAYUJÃ SAKHÃYÃ
SAMÃNAM VRIKŠAM PARI ŠASVAJÃTE
TAYORANYAH PIPALAM SVÃDVATTI
ANSHNAN ANYO ABHI CHÃKSHÎTI (27)

i.e., two friendly, beautiful birds are perched on the same tree. One of them enjoys the fruit of the tree and the other, without eating, watches keenly the accompanying one. The two birds here are God and Soul. The tree is the Nature. Soul enjoys the fruit of Nature, God, without eating, only watches the other's activities. This *Mantra* is the core of the Vedic philosophy can be judged from the fact that the same *Mantra* also appears in the Atharva Veda (9.9.20), the Mundaka Upanishad (3.1.1) and the Svetashvatar Upanishad (4.6). A seal found in the Mohenjo-daro excavations carries the imprint of two birds perched on a tree, testifying the Mohenjo-daro civilisation to belong to the Vedic civilisation (Incidentally, the cover page of this book shows Yoga aspirant meditating under a tree on which two birds are perched).

Thus Spake Plotinus

The Soul and The One are like two concentric circles,
One when they coincide;
And two only when they separate.

24
What is Nature (*Prakriti*) and Its Role

Prakriti is that stuff out of which God creates the Universe. It is the material cause of the Universe. Literally, *Pra* means before and *Kriti* means creation, i.e., the original state of Nature – Primordial Nature, the Holy Grail. This is the first state of *Prakriti* and is defined as SATVA RAJAS TAMASÃM SÃMYÃVASTHÃ PRAKRITIH (64), i.e., *Prakriti* is the state of equilibrium of *Satva*, *Rajas* and *Tamas* – its three *gunas* (traits). *Satva* means Mind/Cognition, *Rajas* means Motion/Activity and *Tamas* means Matter/Stability. *Prakriti's* second state is *Vikriti*, disturbance in the original state; it is the evolutionary stage of creation. Its third state is the created world called *Prãkrit* or *Srišti*. God has created, as it were, everything in triplets – SARVAM TRAI ÃNSHIKAM PÃTÎ (65). *Prakriti* has three constituents – Ãkash (Space), *Kãla* (Time) and *Prãna* (Energy). Space has three dimensions – Length, Width and Depth; Time also has three aspects – Past, Present and Future. Likewise, Energy (Matter) has three forms – Gas, Liquid and Solid.

Prakriti is *sat* (eternal), *Agya* – has no knowledge and *Jada* – inanimate, non-conscious. *Prakriti* is known by many names – *Kšar* (Perishable), *Avyakta* (Unmanifested), *Vykta* (Manisfested), *Drishya* (The Visible), *Kãrana* (Cause – Material Cause), *Pradhãna* (Principal/Main Cause), *Kšetra* (Field), *Sad-asadãtmakam* (Eternal, but changeable). It is *Sat* because it is eternal, it is also *Asat*, because it is changeable. It has been further explained as NÃSHAH KÃRAÑA LAYAH (66), i.e., destruction is dissolution in *Prakriti* (Original State), not annihilation.

This aspect of *Prakriti* (Nature) is known in science by the dictum, 'Matter can neither be created nor be destroyed, it only changes its form'.

Prakriti is also known as *Aditi* (Non-Perishable/Eternal). Rig Veda (1.89.10) elaborates what constitutes *Aditi*:

ADITIR DYAUR ADITIR ANTRIKŠAM
ADITIR MÃTÃ SA PITÃ SA PUTRAH
VISHVEDEVÃ ADITIH PANCH JANA
ADITIR JÃTAM ADITIR JANITVAM (67)

i.e., the heavenly bodies are *Aditi*; the space is *Aditi*; Mother, Father, Son (their bodies) are the product of *Aditi*; all the forces of Nature are *Aditi*; Five elements of Nature and the five Senses are *Aditi*; whatever is born is *Aditi*; the newborn child is *Aditi* and the process of birth is *Aditi*.

Before the creation, *Prakriti* lies in God in a state of stupor, motionless, asleep. At God's will (*Ikšaña*) stirring is created in *Prakriti* and the Universe comes into existence. *Sankhya Darhsana* (1.96) states: TAT SANNIDHÃNÃT ADHIŠTHATRITVAM MAÑIVAT (68), i.e., by the presence of God, a motion is generated in *Prakriti* as does a magnet move pieces of iron in its presence. The Gita (9.10) says:

MAYÃDHYAKŠENA PRAKRITIH
SÛYATE SACHARÃCHARAM
HETUNÃ ANENA KAUNTEYA
JAGAD-VIPARIVARTATE (69)

i.e., O Arjuna! Under my superintendence, *Prakriti* creates this animate and inanimate world. For that reason alone, the cycle of creation keeps moving.

We see from experience in life that whatever is produced or manufactured has a purpose and that it has a user. Now *Prakriti* is *Jada*, inanimate. It is not aware of its existence nor can it use the created things for itself. God is beyond any needs; He also does not use the created things. It is only *Jiva* (Soul) that can make use of created things. So, the purpose of this created world is to serve *Jiva* (Soul). *Sankhya Darshana* (6.40) says ANUPABHOGE-API-PUMARTHAM SRIŠTIH (70), i.e., not using itself, created world (*Prakriti*) is for the use of *Purush* (Soul). *Yoga Darshana* (2.16) also says the same thing: BHOGÃPAVARGÃRTHAM DRISHYAM (71), i.e., the Seen

(Manifested World/*Prakriti*) has its purpose (providing the *Purusha* with), experience (enjoyment of fruits of its action) and liberation. As already stated earlier, Soul cannot act or experience anything except through the medium of a body. *Prakriti* is the material which creates the body and, thereby, helps Soul to undertake its worldly and other worldly pursuits. In short, only Self (Soul) exists for itself (*Svãrtha*); The world of objects exists for another, (*Prãrtha*) the world does not exist of itself.

On Nature

Ether is the mother and reservoir of visible creation
and partaking somehow of the nature of mind.

—Plato

To see a world in a grain of sand
And a heaven in a wild flower
Hold infinity in the palm of your hand
And eternity in an hour.

—William Blake

Galileo saw Nature as a book whose author is God.

—Pope Benedict XVI

The Universe is the mirror of God –
the mirror in which His majesty and perfection are reflected.

—Azim Ibn Mohammad al Nasafi

25
The Doctrine of *Maya* (Illusion)

The *Advaita* Philosohphy (Non-Dualism) has propounded the Doctrine of *Maya*. Their basic tenet is that there exists only one Entity, i.e., *Brahma* (God). They do not believe in the independent entities of Souls or *Prakriti*. Their too-oft quoted tenets define the *Advaita* Philosophy thus: BRAHMA SATYAM JAGAD MITHYÃ (72), i.e., *Brahma* is true; *Jagat* is false – *Brahma* exists, *Jagat* does not; it appears to exist (illusionary). Their second dictum is: JIVO BRAHMETI NETRAH, i.e., *Jiva* (Soul), verily, is *Brahma*, no other. (This issue has already been discussed earlier).

There is a plethora of arguments and counter-arguments on the Doctrine of *Maya*. In short, it runs like this:

(i) The manifested cosmos is the reflection of *Brahma* in *Maya*; the *Jivas* (Souls) are the reflections of *Brahma* in *Avidya*, a part of *Maya*; what remains unaffected is *Ishvara*, says Vachaspati. Strange! The same *Brahma* becomes Three – *Ishvara*, *Jiva* and *Jagat* (Cosmos)! "Now the question arises: does the whole or only a part of *Brahma* change into the world? If it is the whole, then *Brahma* lies before our eyes as the world and there is nothing transcendent which we have to seek. If it is a part that is transformed into the world, then *Brahma* is capable of being partitioned." (Indian Philosophy, Vol. II, page 568 by Dr. S. Radhakrishnan). On this, Swami Vidyanand Saraswati commented thus: "It amounts to cooking half the hen for meals and keeping the other half for laying eggs."

(ii) *Maya* is defined as neither existent nor non-existent, inexplicable. Aditya Purana, quoted by Vijnanabikshu, states:

NA SAD-RÛPÃ NA ASAD-RÛPÃ
MÃYÃ NAIVA-UBHAYÃTMIKÃ
SAD-ASADBHYAM NIRVÃCHYÃ
MITHYÃ-BHÛTÃ SANÃTANÎ (73)

i.e., *Maya* is neither existent nor non-existent, nor is it both combined. The indescribable as either existent or non-existent is of the nature of MITHYA (appearance) and is eternal.

Now, how can a non-existent entity be Eternal? And how can a non-existent entity affect the *Chaitanya-Svarupa* (Pure Consciousness) *Bhrama* and snatch His consciousness and make Him *Jada* (inanimate)? And further, if *Maya* is existent, it appears to be more powerful than the Omnipotent *Brahma* as also it negates the very theory of Non-Dualism.

(iii) *Advaita* believes *Jagat* is *Mithya* (Appearance). Its appearance is likened to the illusion of a snake in a rope. Rope is not a snake but appears like a snake in darkness. Just as appearance of snake is false, the appearance of world is false due to *Maya*. This is known as the theory of VIVARTA (appearance).

Now, it is wrong to say that the serpent does not exist; it does exist and has likeness with a rope which is serpentine. The seer of a rope knows the existence of a snake, in general, and gets frightened. If snake does not exist at all, why does a rope appear like a snake and not a cow or a buffalo? So, the world exists and is real. *Vedanta Darshana* (*Brahma Sutra*) (2.2.27) categorically refutes that the world is false: NA ABHÃVA UPALABDHEH (74), i.e., its non-existence is not proved from the very fact of its availability. The world exists and we enjoy it.

Western Philosopher Richard Bilbur has a penchant dig at the concept of illusion of the world thus:

We milk the cow of the world and as we do
We whisper in her ear, "you are not true."

Guru Nanak assures his disciples:
NANAK SACHE DI SACHI KAAR
SACHA AAP SACHA DARBAR
i.e., Nanak believes that the creation of the true God is true. He is true, His empire is true.

(iv) The Concept of *Maya*, in *Advaita Philosophy*, is illusion, deception (*Prapanch*), but that is not so in the Vedas or the Upanishads. *Maya* in Vedic terminology is synonym of *Prakriti*. Shavetashvatara Upanishad (4.10) says: MÃYÃM TU PRAKRITI VIDYÃT MÃYÃVINAM TU MAHESHVARAM (75), i.e., undoubtedly, regard *Maya* as *Prakriti*; and God as the lord of *Prakriti*. Out of *Prakriti*, God creates this universe.

(v) Thanks to the Doctrine of *Maya*, *Brahma* and *Ishvara* appear to be two different Entities. *Ishvara* is the Lord of the world, but not *Brahma*. In the Vedas and the Upanishads, there is no such distinction. Both the words '*Ishvara*' and '*Brahma*' are synonyms. Rig Veda says: 'EKAM SAT VIPRÃH BAHUDHÃ VADANTI (42)' i.e., God is one; the wise describe Him by many names. *Ishvara*, *Brahma*, *Purusha*, *Atma*, *Parmatma*, *Tat*, *Sat* are all the names of God.

In short, *Maya* is not illusion, but the other name of *Prakriti*.

The Spake Sheikh Sādī

"BARGE DARAKHTĀNE SABZ DAR NAZARE HOSHIĀR
HAR BABQ DAFTARĪST MĀRFATE KARDĪGĀR

In the eyes of a senstive beholder,
Each leaf of a green tree is a
Storehouse of God's workmanship.

26
The Concept of *Trividha* (Three-fold) *Brahma*

The Trinity of God, Souls and Nature has been termed as *Trividha Brahma* in the Shevtashvara Upanishad (1.12):

ETAJ JNEYAM NITYAMEVA ÃTMA-SANSTHAM
NÃTAH PARAM VEDITAVYAM HI KINCHIT
BHOKTA BHOGYAM PRERITÃRAM CHA MATVÃ
SARVAM PROKTAM TRIVIDHAM BRAHMA ETAT (76)

i.e., that Eternal which rests in the Self should be known. Truly, there is nothing beyond this to be known. By knowing the Enjoyer, the Object of Enjoyment and the Mover, everything has been said and that is *Trividha* (Three-fold) *Brahma*.

God, Soul and Nature – all the three are essential for the existence and operation of the universe. And all the three are great. BRIHATVÃT BRAHMA (77), i.e., being great is *Brahma*. As the three entities are indispensible and important, each is great in its own way. All the three despite being different act in unison; that is why, they together are called *Trividha Brahma*. Just as an axel holds and moves the two wheels annexed to it, God is the *Adhishthata* (Matrix) of Soul and Nature.

Let us now examine how the Three act together and are indispensible. Suppose, God and Nature exist, but there is no Soul. Nature, being inanimate, is not conscious of its own existence, nor is it capable of enjoying itself. God is beyond all needs and has no desire to enjoy. In that scenario, all creation will be as futile as goldsmith's ornaments which have no user. In other words, in the absence of Souls, presence of God and Nature will become redundant. Let us now assume there exist God and Souls, but there is no Nature. In that situation,

Souls will be lying in God action-less in perpetuity. Again, God and Souls become redundant. Let us now assume, Souls and Nature exist, but no God. Science affirms that universe was created at some point of time. It has been earlier discussed that neither Nature nor any Soul can create the universe. Here too the two become redundant.

In short, all the three Entities – God, Soul and Nature are essential for the existence and operation of the world and their acting in unison is called Trividha Brahma. Jewish Philosopher Rosenzweig has put the interdependence of the three succinctly thus: "Only when God, the World and Man enter into relationship with one another, they do fully reveal themselves." (Quoted by Dr. S. Radhakrishnan in History of Philosophy: Eastern and Western Voll II Page 92). Korean Philosopher Chun Boe Kynna has expressed the same view about the existence of the three Entities thus, "The one that is visible (manifested world) begins from the invisible (Primordial Nature/The Holy Grail). The Invisible consists of three Ultimates and their essence is infinite."

Even scanning of the names of God in the Vedic literature reveals existence of the three Entities. Names like AUM, SVAYAMBHU (SELF- BORN), SACHIDANADA (Eternal, Pure Consciousness, Bliss) denote God alone. Names like JAGAD-AMBA (Mother of the Universe), HIRANYA-GARBHA (Womb of Heavenly Bodies), SRISHTI-KARTA (Creator of the Universe) point to the existence of Nature, apart from Him. And names like 'SA NO BANDHUR JANITÃ SA VIDHÃTÃ (78), i.e., He is our Brother, Father and Ruler point to the existence of Souls other than Himself. He cannot be brother, father or ruler of Himself. In short, there are three entities – *Ishvara*, *Jiva*, *Prakriti*.

Trividha Brahma (The Divine Trinity) not only exists, it is reflected in our day-to-day activities. For example, while we are very happy, we unknowingly utter 'Ha! Ha! Ha!' (Thrice). When we are in a hurry, we unknowingly say 'Run, Run, Run' (Thrice). Can any Biologist or Psychologist explain why such utterances are automatically uttered thrice and not four times? During games and sports in schools and colleges as also in Olympic Games, the concerned organiser pronounces, 'One, Two, Three,' or 'Ready, Steady, Go' and the game starts. Why does the game start at the pronouncement of the word 'Three'? Has any Code of Conduct been issued in this regard? No. Further, at an auction, when the Bid amount is repeated thrice, the Bid becomes final and legal. Any bid thereafter is illegal. Can any expert of Jurisprudence explain what accords legal sanctity to the Bid announced thrice? At any religious ceremony, the name of God 'Aum' or famous Gayatri Mantra is chanted either once or thrice. If it is chanted once, the devotee is bowing to or acknowledging the presence of God; if thrice, he is acknowledging the presence of *Trividha Brahma*, the Divine Trinity.

Jewish View On Trinity

All things of which this world consists,
spirits as well as bodies will return to their Principal,
the root from which they proceeded.
—Jewish Mystic Book : Zohar

W.D. Brown On Vedic Religion

"It recognizes but One God. It is a thoroughly scientific religion where religion and science meet hand in hand. Here theology is based upon science and philosophy".
—The Superiority of Vedic Religion

27
The Doctrine of *Karma*

Given below are the salient features of The Doctrine of *Karma*:

Karma is the the *Dharma* of *Jiva*.

There is no English equivalent of the Sanskrit word '*Karma*'. All the same, *Karma* means Action, Deed or Activity which is done physically, mentally or orally. Similarly, *Dharma* has no equivalent English word. *Dharma* means natural trait or tendency as Fire has the natural trait to give light and heat. *Dharma* means duty, e.g., the duty of a father, a teacher, a solider or a ruler; *Dharma* means ethical, moral and spiritual values: *Dharma* is not Religion, but the core (ethical, moral, spiritual values) of every religion, devoid of form, is *Dharma*. George Bernard Shaw rightly said, "Religion is one, though there are hundreds of branches of it." That Religion is *Dharma*.

So, *Karma* is the natural trait of *Jiva*. The Vedic definition of *Jiva* is KRATUMAYAH PURUŠAH (79), i.e., *Purusha* (*Jiva*/Soul) is active. Science also says the same thing: "Activity is the manifestation of life." But, the peculiarity of The Doctrine of *Karma* is that it is only Man (Homo Sapiens) who acts. All other species (Souls in other life-forms) do not perform any *Karma*; they perform only activities or instinctive actions, assigned to them. Human Beings are called *Karma Yoni*, all other life-forms are *Bhog Yoni*: it is not that Souls in other species have not performed '*Karmas*', they had but in their previous lives, the fruits/punishment for which they are undergoing now.

What is the specialty of Human Beings that only they can perform *Karma*? *Nirukta* (3.8.2) poses and answers this question:

MANUŠYÃH KASMÃT MATVÃ KARMÃÑI SÎVAYANTI (80), i.e., why are they called Men? Because they juxtapose their actions with their intellect. Modern science also regards man as rational being. God has bestowed man with intellect to analyse things, assess pros and cons and decide and act one way or the other. He has the freedom of choice. Hence, he becomes responsible for his actions – *Karma*. All other species have no such choice or freedom.

Karma and its fruits

The basic tenet of The Doctrine of *Karma* is that every action has its fruit. There is an Upanishadic saying: 'AVASHYAMEVA HI BHOGTAVYAM KRITAM KARMA SHUBHA ASHUBHAM' (81) i.e., one must reap the fruit of one's good or bad deeds. One must get reward or punishment of one's good or bad deeds in this life or next or after hundreds or thousands of lives. No deed vanishes without fruit. Goswanmi Tulsidas has said:

KARMA PRADHÃN VISHA RACHI RÃKHÃ
JO JAS KARAHIN SO TAS FAL CHÃKHÃ
i.e., God has designed the world such
As one does, so does one reap its fruit.

While detailed discussion on this subject is penned in the following pages, I am impelled to quote a historicl factual incident (Source: Social Media) which amply illustrates how good deeds fructify and yield good results. One farmer in England, by the name of Flemming, saw a child in a terrible condition and saved his life. The father of that child visited Flemming's house in the evening and offered him a huge sum as reward for saving his son's life. Flemming refused to accept this, saying that it was his duty to save the child. The visitor was deeply impressed by this reply. In the meantime, a child came out of Flemming's hut. On knowing that the child was Flemming's son, the visitor offered to take care of his son's education with the observation that with the inheritance of his father's values and with proper education, his son, one day, will become a great man. Flemming accepted this offer with thanks. The gentleman kept his promise and educated this child like his own son. This child became a renowned scientist - Alexander Flemming who invented pencillin vaccine which saved lives of millions! The gentleman who sponsored his education was Rudolf Churchill. And the child whose life farmer Flemming had saved, later came to be known as Sir Winston Churchill!

In Indian Philosophy, God is known as Karmâdhyakša, one who dispenses justice as per the karmas of individual souls. God's Law of Karma works incessantly but no one knows when someone's action gets fructified. Leo Tolstoy's story 'God Sees the Truth but Waits' also illustrates this point. As per this story, a murderer who becomes a fugitive and lives in the garb of a 'saint' gets caught and punished for a murder which he did not commit, but breaks down and admits the murder he committed 20 years ago!

Soul Has Only The Right to Act

The other important tenet of The Doctrine of *Karma* is that Soul has the right only to act, but not over its fruit. The Gita's central advice is: (2.47)

KARMAÑYEVA ADHIKÃRASTE
MÃ FALEŠU KADÃCHANA
MÃ KARMAFALA-HETURBHÛR
MÃ TE SANGO AKARMAÑI (82)

i.e., to action alone hast thou right and never at all to its fruits. Let not the fruits of action be thy motive; neither let there be in thee any attachment to inaction (Translation by Dr. S. Radhakrishnan). Man's right and freedom to act has already been explained above; but why has he no right over the fruit? It does not mean that he will not get its fruit, he certainly will; but not as he wishes, and justifiably so. If a student appears in an examination, he cannot be expected to assess his own performance. First, he does not have the capacity to do so e.g., answer to which question is right and which wrong. Second, if he is given the authority to do so, his judgement will be favourably biased. A criminal cannot be allowed to sit in judgement over his crime, for obvious reasons. Furthermore, there are many other factors and circumstances which play a role in God's judgement of which we cannot be aware. So, the advice is one should not be obsessed with the fruit of one's action. This advice is coupled with the other advice of not harbouring the feeling if I am not going to get fruit as I desire, why should I act, better not toil and sit idle. No. One should not adopt this course, because inaction is also action, an act of omission. Furthermore, the Gita (3.5) says:

NAHI KASHCHIT-KŠANAM-API
JÃTU TIŠTHATY-AKARMA-KRIT (83)

i.e., for no one can remain, even for a moment, without doing work.

28

The Gita's Views on *Karma*, *Akarma*, *Vikarma*

As one is responsible for one's actions, one should be very alert about what one does. The Gita has advised us to be morally alert and properly scrutinise what is *Karma* (action), what is the *Akarma* (inaction) and what is *Vikarama* (wrong action). The Gita (4.18) specifically advises:

KARMAÑY AKARMA YAH PASHYED
AKARMAÑI CHA KARMA YAH
SA BUDDHIMÃN MANUŠYEŠU
SA YUKTAH KRITSANA-KARMA KRIT (84)

i.e., he who in action sees inaction and action in inaction, he is wise among men. He is a Yogi and he has accomplished all his work. How? One who discriminates between good or bad, virtue or vice is wise, but one who does not is *Dharmavimud*, spiritually blind. To illustrate our point, we recall an incident in our history. Prithvi Raj Chauhan in a battle with Mohammed Gauri laid down his arms to avoid the sin of killing cows arraigned before the enemy's army. In this *Karma* – In the act of laying down his arms, he failed to discern his *Akarma*, inaction to fight his enemy and, thereby, by vicarious responsibility, became responsible for the *Vikrama*, heinous deeds of massacre and plunder, including the killing of the cows which his spiritual blindness (*Dharmavimud*) intended to protect. Similarly, if a soldier deployed at a border-post leaves it unattended to say prayer or read Namaz at the appointed time, is committing an *Akarma* (not attending, the post duty) and may be committing *Vikarma*, if attacked by the enemy, observing the post unattended.

Karma and Character

The other important feature of The Doctrine of *Karma* is that one's *Karmas* determine one's character or Nature. Whatever one does, thinks or utters leaves an impression on one's mind as does one leave an imprint of one's footsteps on sand after treading on it. This is called *Sanskara*. Take a handful of rose-petals, keep these for a few moments and throw these away. This act will leave some odour in your palm which you can still enjoy. The tendency to repeat this act of enjoying the sweet smell again is called *Vasana*. One's good and bad actions leave *Sanskara* in one's mind that generate *Vasana* or propensity to repeat the actions that leads to formation of one's nature or character. That is why some people are calm and kind, some cruel and ferocious; some fun-loving, some serious and studious, some alcoholic and some compulsive gamblers or smokers. But situation is not frustrating or defeating. The situation can be changed by *Shiksha* and *Diksha*, i.e., by counselling, training and efforts. Here comes the role of will power and freedom. Sage Charaka says: SANSKÃRO HI GUÑÃNTAR-ÃDHÃNAM UCHAYATE (85), i.e., verily, imbibing different traits is called *Sanskara*.

The following statements of some great philosophers will guide us how *Karma* and Character are intricately interconnected:

"Watch your thoughts, they become your words.
Watch your words, they became your actions.
Watch your actions, they become your habits.
Watch you habits, they became your character.
Watch your character, for it will become you destiny."

— Frank Outlaw

"We are what we repeatedly do. Men acquire a particular quality by constantly acting in a particular way. You become just by performing just actions, temperate by performing temperate actions, brave by performing brave actions."

— Aristotle

"We are every moment making our characters and shaping our destinies... Sin is not so much a defiance of God as a denial of Soul; not so much a violation of law as a betrayal of Self."

— Dr. S. Radhakrishnan (The Hindu View of Life, Page 52-53)

29

Karma and Destiny (*Bhgaya*)

At times, some happenings in life make one doubt the theory of *Karma* and one starts believing that *Bhagya* or Destiny is more important and convincing. For example, one gets an amount of crores of rupees in a lottery without any effort to deserve such a big amount. Or during construction of a house, one digs up a pot containing old gold coins, again by freak of luck. Conversely, a student who has worked hard and is extremely intelligent falls sick on the examination day and wastes a year. Worse still, a son of an old man, who has acquired PhD., MD. or M.Tech degree suddenly dies in a road accident without enjoying the fruit of his hard work and depriving his parents of any help in old age. If all this is not bad luck, fate, destiny or *Durbhagya*, what else?

When the Gita says (as mentioned earlier) that you do not have any authority to get the fruit for your action, it does not mean that the fruit you get will be arbitrarily decided by God, the *Karmadhyaksha*. There are certain imponderables like the past life *karmas* and factors which go into the fruit, of which we are not aware. Only God knows what fruit of which action will be dispensed when. Dr. S. Radhakrishnan states in his book 'The Hindu View of life', "The Principle of *Karma* insists on the primacy of the ethical and identified God with the rule of law. All is law, yet all's God. *Karma* is not a mechanical principle but a spiritual necessity. It is the embodiment of the mind and will of God. God is the supervisor, *Karmadhyaksha*."

All the above incidents though appear to be unrelated with any action of the person concerned in this life, but he carries a baggage of innumerable/previous lives. Such occurrences are the fruit of his actions/*Karmas* in previous lives.

The following verse of Mahãbhãratã (*Anushãsan Parva*) replies categorically to the doubts raised above:

KEVALAM GRAHA-NAKSTRAM
NA KAROTI SHUBHÃSHUBHAH
SARVAM ÃTMAKRITAM KARMA
LOKAVÃDO GRAHÃ ITI (86)

It is not the stars that bring good or bad fortune, people call all the *Karmas* done by the Self in the past as stars' effect.

In the Mahãbhãratã, Duryodhana blames some godly power for his undesirable deeds. He says:

JÃNÃMI DHARMAM NA CHA ME PRAVRITTIH
JÃNÃMI ADHARMAM NA CHA ME NIVRITTIH
KENÃPI DEVENA HRIDI STHITENA
YATHÃ NIYUKTO ASMI TATHÃ KAROMI. (87)

i.e., i know what is right, but I do not have the propensity to do the same. I know what it wrong, but I cannot refrain from it. By some godly power, sitting in me, as I am dictated, so I act. What Duryodhana is referring to as godly power is nothing but his own altered ego developed by repeated wrong deeds and distorted thinking, mentioned in the Subsection *Karma* and Character. Shakespeare's following words in Julius Caesar are relevant in this context:

Fault, Dear Brutus, is not in our stars
But in ourselves that we are underlings.

It is Duryodhana's own moral bankruptcy that in goading him to do more such immoral acts.

Rudyard Kipling's words are also very relevant in this context: "If your being is right, you cannot possibly go wrong." Blaming the stars or some other power is only an alibi.

The Doctrine of *Karma* is both spiritual and scientific. There are only two entities who know everything you do, think or utter. One, yourself and the other God, who is seated in you. The modern generation will understand better God's functioning by the analogy of a computer. God is like a Divine Super Computer who is registering everything you do; His software of Rita and Satya (explained earlier) works out the quantum of reward or punishment based on one's deeds of which He is Himself a witness, being Omnipresent. Just as a rocket with precise software follows the designated path and reaches the determined destination, say, Moon or Mars, similarly the Divine software lands the

Souls in the specified species or places. The *Shãnkhãyana Ãranyaka* (3.2) says SA IH STHÃNEŠU PRATYÃJÃYATE YATHÃ KARMA YATHÃ VIDYAM (88), i.e., *Jiva* (Soul) takes birth in life-form or place (country) as per his deeds and level of knowledge. God, the Divine Super Computer, is installed in the Soul itself and takes him to the designated *Yoni* or place. Neither chance nor stars have any role in it. Nor the choice of the Souls concerned matters. Obviously, no one would like to be born as a snake or a scorpio.

Classification of *Karmas*

Karmas are of three types – Virtuous (*Punya*), Sins (*Paap*) and Mishrits (*Mixed*). These are classified in three categories – *Kriyamãn* (Present Deeds), *Sanchit* (Accumulated) and *Prãrabadha* (Fructified).

There are certain deeds which fructify immediately. If you put a burning coal on your palm, the result will be instant. Some actions take time to fructify, e.g., if you plant a mango tree, you will have to wait for five to six years to taste its fruit. Some actions may not fructify in one's life time. Only God knows which *Karmas* fructify when. The action we perform at present is called *Kriyaman Karma*. If its fruit is given, it gets exhausted. The deeds the fruits of which we do not get at present are accumulated and are called *Sanchit Karma*. It is like a bank balance. These lie in the Sukshma *sharira* (Astral Body). When, under the design of God, the deeds that become ripe for fruition, we call *Prarabadha*. When a Soul takes birth, its *Prarabadha* decides which life-form it will acquire, how long will it live in that body and what pains and pleasures it will experience. If it is born a human being, the present deeds which do not fructify will be added to the *Sanchit* – the Reservoir of *Karmas*. Thus, this cycle continues.

Now which actions earn a Soul human birth and which actions are responsible for animal or insect-forms, only God knows. However, in Manusmiriti (12.40, 12.9), in the Puranas and other scriptures, there are some descriptions:

DEVATVAM SÃTVIKÃ YÃNTI
MANUŠYATVAM CHA RÃJASÃH
TIRYAKTVAM TÃMSÃ
NITYAM-ITYEŠA TRIVIDHÃ GATIH (89)

SHARÎRJAIH KARMA DOSAIR
YÃTI STHÃVARATÃM NARAH
VÃCHIKAIH PAKŠÎMRIGATÃM
MÃNSAIR ANTYA JÃTITÃM (90)

i.e., souls with noble deeds are born as saints, sages, geniuses; Souls with deeds of *Rajas* qualities are born as ordinary human beings, Souls with deeds of *Tamas* qualities are born in lower forms such as insects. These are the three channels of birth. Those who commit sins physically, e.g., murder, theft, etc. get birth as trees and vegetation; those who commit sins orally are born as birds and animals; those who commit sins mentally are born as lower human beings like butcher.

Just as in a prison, a prisoner is made to do hard work, e.g., breaking bricks or weaving baskets, similarly Soul taking birth in flora and fauna forms, not only suffer heat and cold or rain and gale in the open, they also bear delicious fruits and nutritious vegetables to serve others. Insects also maintain ecological balance. Frogs, for example, are useful for making the land fertile. So, their sins are getting mitigated, under the design of God and they get back human form after some innumerable births in these forms. Heraditus has righty said, "God no doubt, is the embodiment of Cosmic Justice."

While only God knows what punishments He awards for different kinds of sins, it is interesting to note similarity of views of Greek philosopher Plotinus with those of Manu, cited above:

"Those who have sought only to gratify their lust and appetite pass into the bodies of lascivious and gluttonous animals. Those who have degraded their senses by disuse are compelled to vegetate in the plants. Those who have ruled tyrannically become eagles. He who has acquired civil virtues becomes a man. If he does not have these virtues, he it transformed into a domestic animal like a bee."

– Plotinus (The Case for the Reincarnation, – Joe Fisher)

30
Non-Hindu Sciptures' and Philosophers' View on *Karma*

I. Good and evil do not wrongly befall men;
But Heaven sends down misery or
Happiness according to their conduct.

—Confucius (Luki 39.18)

II. The recompense of good and evil
Follows as the shadow follows figure.

—Tao (Tai Shang Kan Yieng Pien)

III. If a man speaks or acts with evil thought
Pain surely follows him, even as the wheel
Follows the ox that drags the cart along.

—Buddhist Maha Vagga (6.31.7)

IV. Those evil ones, the hateful, cruel, mean
Fall into evil wombs, birth after birth
Till by reaction consequent, in pain
They learn to turn into the ways of good.

—Zoroastrian Scripture Gatha (5.1.6)

(Quoted in the Essential Unity of All Religions:
Bhagvan Dass 'Bharat Ratna')

V. To him that sowest righteousness, shall be a sure reward
Men do not gather grapes of thorns or figs of thistles.
The wage of sin is death... God will render to everyone
According to his deeds.

—The Holy Bible

VI. Those deeds of yours shall verily be brought
Back unto you, as if you were yourself
The author of your own just punishment.

—Hadis: Sayings of Prophet Mohammed

VII. *Karma* is the law of spiritual gravitation.

— A.E. Russell

VIII. "In the long run, everyone will pay the penalty of his own misdeeds. The man who remembers this will be angry with no one, revile no one, hate no one."

—Epictetus

Umar Bine Hash-shâm's Wish

VA SAHABI KEYÃM FEMAKÃMIL HINDE YAUMANA
VA YAQULÛNA LÃTAHAZANA FINNAKA TAVAJJARÛ

—Umar Bine Hash-shâm (Uncle of Prophet Mohammad)
SE ARUL OKÛL Page 235

"O God! Take away my whole life, grant me only one day's stay in India, because having reached there, man attains liberation."

31
The Doctrine of Reincarnation of Soul

To take birth after death is called reincarnation or transmigration of Soul, but why at all this phenomenon should take place? We now explain why does Soul take birth again and again; what are the proofs to prove reincarnation of Soul and what are the views of different religions or renowned philosophers on this issue.

Karma and Reincarnation

We have already explained that one must reap the fruits of one's good or bad deeds. Experience tells us that it is not possible to reap fruits of all one's deeds in one lifetime. Furthermore, for one murder, one can be hanged once; for two murders or multiple murders also one can be hanged once. To emphasise the gravity of multiple murders, the criminals in the west have been awarded imprisonment up to 400 years, which is impossible to undergo. There are also instances of suicide bombers who kill scores of men and escape the clutches of law. How can they be punished? The Vedic solution is rebirth of the criminal to undergo punishment in the next life/lives. The Upanishadic dictum is:

NÃBHUKTAM KSIYATE KARMA
JANMAKOTISHATAIRAPI (91)

i.e., no deed gets exhausted without fructification even in hundreds of crores (billions) of birth.

The Doctrine of Karma and the Doctrine of Reincarnation of Soul are interconnected. As one is unable to reap the fruits of one's deeds in one life, the unspent-up deeds are carried forward in the next life. At birth, whatever one brings along is called *Prarabdha* (literally, to begin with, the opening balance). The following words of Dastur

Khurshid Dabu, the High Priest of Parsi Fire Temple, Bombay, are pertinent in this regard:

"If God's arithmetic and book-keeping are correct, then there is some balance brought forward from the previous account."

When that opening balance, along with the disposable *Karma* of this life, are spent up, the Soul moves on for the next birth. Mahabharata (Anushasan Parva) says: TIŠTHET KARMA FALAM YÃVAT VRAJET KARMA KŠAYE PUNAH (92), i.e., Soul stays in this body till it reaps the designated fruit and takes up the journey for the annihilation of other *Karmas* by reaping their fruit.

Thus Spake a Sufi Poet

RUH AUR JISM KÃ RISHTÃ BHI AJAB HAI
SÃRÎ UMAR SÃTH RAHE LEKIN TUÃRUF NÃ HUVÃ

Strange is the relationship between Soul and Body!
Lived together the whole life
And yet did not get introduced to each other!

32
Proofs of Soul's Reincarnation

(i) Scriptural Evidences

There are scriptural evidences about the re-birth of **Soul.** Yajur Veda (4.15) says

PUNAR MANAH PUNAR ÃYURMA ÃGAN
PUNAH PRÃÑAH PUNAR ÃTMÃ MA ÃGAN
PUNAH CHAKŠUH PUNAH SHROTRAM MA ÃGAN
VAISHVÃNARO ADABDHAS TANÛPÃ
AGNIR NAH PÃTU DURITÃDAVADYÃT (93)

i.e., O God! At each birth, give us pure mind, long life, vitality, pure Soul, sound eyes and ears. O Ruler of the World! Nourish our bodies in all our life-terms and save us from misery and misdeeds. The Vedic grammar Nirukta (13.19) declares:

MRITASHCHÃHAM PUNARJÃTO
JÃTASHCHÃHAM PUNARMRITAH
NÃNÃYONI SAHASRÃÑI
MAYOŠITÃNI YÃNI VAI (94)

i.e., after death, I was born again; After taking birth, I died again. I have utilised thousands of wombs of different species. Saint Augustine is expressing the same sentiment by posing question to himself, "Did I not live in another body before entering my mother's womb?" The Gita (2.27) categorically declares:

JÃTASYA HI DHRUVO MRITUR
DHRUVAM JANMA MRITASYA CHA (95)

i.e., for the one that is born, death is certain and certain is birth for the one that has died.

(ii) Proof of Disparities at Birth

All the religions of the world believe that God is Kind, Just and Merciful. Everybody takes birth at the will of God. We see in life, some are born in rich families, some are born to parents living in abject poverty; some are born beautiful and some ugly; some are born healthy and some are born handicapped; some are born geniuses and some imbeciles. The newborn have not done any wrong or committed any sin or any virtuous deeds, for which they have been rewarded or punished. If there is no previous life in which they must have performed good or bad deeds, then God will turn out to be unkind, unjust and unmerciful.

Furthermore, it is difficult to explain for child prodigies. Some children at young age are known to have exhibited extraordinary talent in music, painting or mathematics. For Mozart could play piano at the age of four; Pascal could solve problems of plain geometry and calculus at the age of ten; Ramanujan became world-renowned mathematician without getting any formal education. Still further, renowned spiritual giants like Mahatma Buddha, Shankaracharya, Swami Dayanand, Swami Vivekanand, geniuses like Shakespeare, Kalidas, Einstein were all born of ordinary parents, where did they get their extraordinary spiritual, literary or scientific acumen? One has to believe they must have developed these faculties in their earlier lives.

(iii) Instances of Memories of Previous Lives

There have been numerous instances of small children of the age of 3-10 who exhibited memories of previous lives. Their utterances with regard to the place, parents and recurrences of previous birth were found to be true. Dr. Ian Stevenson has investigated hundreds of such cases of memories of previous birth and found those to be true. His statement is worthy of attention, "Further investigation of apparent memories of former incarnations may well establish reincarnation as the most probable explanation of those experiences."

One unique feature of incidents of memories of previous life is that these well-up in children of small age who died in an accident or in other tragic and traumatic circumstances in previous lives. This phenomenon which has been noticed by the investigators like Ian Stevenson finds mention in the Mahabharata (*Shasan Parva*):

YE MRITÃH SAHASÃ MARTYÃH
JÃYANTE SAHASÃ PUNAH
TEŠÃM PAURÃÑIKO BHÃVAH
KINCHIT KÃLAM HI TIŠTHTI (96)

i.e., those who dic suddenly and are born again immediately, their old experiences (memories) stay for a short duration. It is further stated that memory of such '*Jãti-Smarah*' persons with memory of previous birth vanishes like a dream as they grow up.

Researches into the phenomenon of reincarnation revealed that some totally illiterate people who have studied no foreign language in this life could, in a state of trance or fit of unconsciousness, interpret passages of foreign classical languages. Dr. Novil Vimaun conducted numerous experiments on illiterate American medium George Valentine who translated passages of Sanskrit, Arabi, Persian, Greek and Chinese languages. Similarly, an English girl Rosemary could pronounce sounds of ancient Egyptian language, Hieroglyphs, on the basis of which Dr. Frederick Wood compiled a Rosemary Egypitian Dictionary. Dr. A.W. Osborne in his book 'The Super Physical' stated: "Dr. Frederick Wood considers that this case provides the strongest inference of immortality hitherto published in evidential form."

Commenting on these incidents, Dr. Ian Stevenson has stated that from these instances, there could be two inferences: either the spirit of a deceased person gripped these persons or these are cases of reincarnation. To us these appear to be cases of reincarnation of Souls who learnt these languages in previous incarnations. Even if some disincarnate spirits entered their bodies and interpreted unknown foreign languages, it stands proved that Souls, after death, carry experiences in the next life. That being established, the possibility of these experiences getting welled-up in the future lives cannot be ruled out.

(iv) Proof of Instinctive Behaviour

Our instinctive behaviour is a potent proof of re-birth. The following existences are indicative of this:

a. At times, we meet a person for the first time and we start liking or disliking him. We do not know anything about him, have never had any interactions with him and still it happens. It is indicative of interaction with him in the past life. While Sir Walter Scott makes a mention in his diary in 1828 that it appears that the persons he was talking to had talked with him in some previous life, John Gay puts it poetically thus:

   "We only part to meet again;
   Change, as ye list, ye winds,
   My heart shall be
   The faithful compass that
   Still points to thee."

b. A newly born human child or a cow's calf starts sucking milk from his mother's breast. Nyaya Darshana (3.1.22) explains:

   PRETYA AHÃRA ABHYÃSA KRITÃT STANY ABHILÃŠAT (97), i.e., a newborn's desire to suck breast is due to previous birth's feeding experience. Similarly, a newborn fish starts swimming and a newborn bird on getting wings flies in the sky. Who gives them the training? They got this training in the previous births.

c. A mouse seeing a cat runs for shelter; a deer seeing a lion, runs fast to save life; birds perched on a tree fly away at the sound of a stone-throw or a gun-shot. All are afraid of death; yet none has experienced death in this life. This fear of death was gained by them in previous lives.

d. A newborn child, without any visible cause, is seen smiling, crying or trembling with fear. Nyaya Darshan (3.1.19) explains this phenomenon thus:

PÛRVA-ABHYASTA-SMRITY-ANUBANDHÃJ JÃTASYA HARŠ-BHAYA-SHOKA-SAMPRATI PATTEH (98)
i.e., the newborn experiences happiness, fear and sorrow owing to his remembrances of the past lives. In this context, William Wordsworth's 'Ode to Intimation of Immortality' is worth reading:

"Our birth is but a sleep and a forgetting
To Soul that rises with us, our life's star,
Hath had elsewhere setting...
Heaven lies around us in our infancy!
Shades of prison-house begin to close upon the growing boy."

Thus Spake Aldous Huxley

"No Self can go beyond the limits of selfhood, either morally
(by the practice of the virtues that brake attachment)
or mystically
(by direct cognitive union with the Ultimate Reality),
unless it is fully aware of what it is and why it is what it is.
Self-transcendence is through self-consciousness"

33
Views of Renowned Philosophers on Reincarnation of Soul

"Without successive lives, life in the universe will disappear."

—Socrates

"Our Souls existed formerly apart from our bodies. The Souls of the dead must exit somewhere whence they came into being again, for the Soul is strong enough by nature to endure coming into being many times."

—Plato

"There is no death of anyone, but only in appearance, even as there is no birth of anyone, save only in seeming. The change from being to becoming seems to be birth and change from becoming to being seems to be death; but, in reality, no one is ever born, nor does one ever die."

—Appollonious of Tyana

"Birth is not a beginning; death is not an end."

—Chauang Tzu

"How come one person is born a genius and another a boob; one is born beautiful and another ugly; one is born healthy and another crippled? The concept of rebirth on earth would enable us to believe there is justice in the Universe."

—C.J. Ducasse

"A tomb is not a blind alley; it is a thoroughfare. It closes on the twilight. It opens on the dawn."

—Victor Hugo

"After all, it is no more surprising to be born twice than to be born once."

— F.M.A. Voltaire

"Every newborn being indeed comes fresh and blithe into the new existence, and enjoys it as a free gift; but there is, and can be, nothing freely given. Its fresh existence is paid for by the old age and death of a worn-out existence which has perished, but which contained the indestructible seed-out of which this new existence has arisen: they are being."

— Arthur Schopenhauer

"The most promising evidence bearing on reincarnation seems to come from the spontaneous cases, especially among children. Often a child begins fumbling at the age of two or even less to communicate his memories of a previous life."

— Ian Stevenson

"If you were to destroy in mankind the belief is immortality, not only love but every living force maintaining the life of the world would at once be dried up. Moreover, nothing then would be immortal, everything would be permissible, even cannibalism."

— Fedor Dostoyevsky

"There is no doubt that through our actions, we are trying to achieve perfection and to remove imperfections. If our world is based on a just and moral order, then it is imperative that we should one day achieve this goal. But most people whom we know are not able to achieve this goal in one life. Therefore, it is only logical for us to believe that there must be a life after this life, so that we can achieve this goal. Otherwise, we have to give up our faith in justice, order and perfection."

— Immanuel Kant

"As to your life, I reckon you are the leavings of many deaths. No doubt, I myself have died thousand times before."

— Walt Whitman

"Who toiled a slave may come anew a prince,
For gentleness and merit won.
Who ruled a prince may wander earth in rags
For things done or undone."

— Sir Edwin Arnold

All things are but altered. Nothing dies
And here and there the unbodied soul flies,
By Time or force or sickness dispossessed
And lodges where it lights in man or beast.

— Pythagoras

"I lived in the Judea eighteen centuries ago... As far back as I can remember, I have unconsciously referred to the experiences of a previous state of existence."

— Thoreau

"I hold that when a person dies
His Soul returns again to earth.
Arrayed in some new flesh disguise;
Another mother gives him birth
With sturdier limits and brighter brain.
The old Soul takes the road again."

— John Masefield, England's Poet Laureate

"It is conceivable that I might be reborn as a Chinese coolie.
In that case, I should lodge a protest."

— Sir Winston Churchill

"To reject the old frame and to assume a new body is inevitable."

— Moshang (Zoroastrianism)

"I should like to be reborn seven times into this world of men so I might destroy the enemies of the court (of Emperor Godrigo)."

— Dying wish of Kusunoki Masashige, a Japanese Commander in 1336 AD

"Belief in reincarnation has existed for thousands of years, and concept has flourished at one time or another in virtually every part of the world. Roughly two-thirds of the world's modern population accepts some form of reincarnation or rebirth as fundamental belief, most notably Hindus and Buddhists as well as many tribal societies. Western belief in reincarnation is low, but has slowly increased since the late 19th century."

In the 20th century, belief in reincarnation has spread fairly evenly throughout the predominantly Christian West, according to the few public opinion polls that have been taken.

In 1969, a George Gallop Poll of adults in twelve countries showed that belief in reincarnation ranged from a low of 10% (The Netherlands) to a high of 26% (Canada). The United States registered

20%, while the United Kingdom scored 18%. Roughly one quarter of those in major religious denominations said they were believers: 26% of Methodists, 25% of Catholics, 22% of Lutherans and 21% of Protestants.

Throughout the Pacific Island Cultures, reincarnation also holds strong. It is found among Balinese, Okainawas Ainu (Northern Japan), Tasmanians (Australia), Morris (New Zealand), Fijians and the inhabitants of New Caledonia, Solomon Islands and Malenesia. In North America, many native American tribes believe in reincarnation. Reincarnation belief also exists among the Native Central and South Americans. "In Africa, believes of rebirth of the human Soul as non-human are more commonplace than human to human rebirth believes. Non-Human forms include animals, birds, reptiles, insects, plants and fabulous monsters."

— Encyclopaedia of Mystical and Paranormal Experience
(Pages 500-504)
Rosemary Ellen Guiley

Thus Spake Epictetus

"There is but one way to tranquillity of mind and happiness:
let this, therefore, be always ready at hand with thee,
both when thou wakest early in the morning
and all the day long, and when thou goest late to sleep,
to account no external things thine own,
but commit all these to God."

34
References of Reincarnation in Non-Hindu Religions

Adherents of Buddhism, Jainism, Sikhism and Zoroastrianism (Parsis) as also ancient Jewish, Chinese and Egyptian civilisations believe in Reincarnation, but majority of the modern adherents of Judaism, Christianity and Islam have no faith in Reincarnation. Some Western scholars believe that the Holy Bible, The Holy Quran and the Judaic scriptures contain references about the concept of Reincarnation. Their views are given below verbatim:

Christianity

1. "Reincarnation is assumed in the Bible teaching."

   — Dictionary of all Scriptures and Myths
2. "Put not off from day to day and from cycle to cycle, in the belief that ye will succeed in obtaining the mysteries when ye return to the world in another cycle."

   — Jesus Christ (from the Gnostic Scripture, Pistis Sophia)
3. "Souls are poured one into another of different kinds of bodies of the world."

   — (Jesus to Magdalene Gnostic Gospel Pistis Sophia)
4. Several of most explicit statements are made by Jesus Christ who affirmed his own pre-existence with the words:
   "Before Abraham was, I am." (John 8.58)
5. In the Gospel, according to Mathew, chapter XI, Jesus identifies John the Baptist as being Elijah reborn.
   (All the above are quoted in The Case for Reincarnation by Joe Fisher.)

6. No honest theologian can, therefore, deny that his acceptance of Jesus as Christ logically binds every Christian to a belief in reincarnation, in Elijah case, at least.

   — Robert Graves

7. Reincarnational teaching in the Bible is largely 'taken for granted, cropping out here and there as a fundamental rock', to quote from E.D. Walker's classic nineteenth-century work Reincarnation. Several Biblical passages only make sense if they are interpreted in the context of repeated Earth lives. The following New Testament extract is one of several allusions to the same kind of hard-fought struggle for the godhead as that envisaged by the Hindus and Buddhists:

   "Him that overcometh will I make a pillar in the temple of my God, and he shall go no more out."

   — (Revelation 3.12)

   [Quoted in The Case for Reincarnation Page 90 – Joe Fisher]

   The aforesaid extract from the Holy Bible has a striking similarity with the Gita (15.6) :

   YADGATVÃ NA NIVARTANTE
   TADDHÃMA PARAMAM MAMA (99)

   i.e., Having reached where do not return, that resort is my Eternal Home.

8. There were indeed references to reincarnation in the Old and the New Testaments. In A.D. 325, the Roman emperor Constantine the Great, along with his mother, Helena, had deleted references to reincarnation contained in the New Testament. The second Council of Constantinople, meeting in A.D. 553 confirmed this action and declared the Concept of Reincarnation a heresy. Apparently, they thought this concept would weaken the growing power of the Church by giving humans too much time to seek their salvation. Yet the original references had been there; the early Church Fathers had accepted the concept of reincarnation. The early Gnostics – Clement of Alexandria, Origen, Saint Jerome, and many others – believed that they had lived before and would again.

   — Dr. Brian Weiss (Many Lives Many Masters, Pages 35-36

Judaism

9. The wellspring of Judaism's esoteric mysticism is the Kabala and that is where reincarnation or gilgul, the Hebrew for 'circuit' or 'rotation' is to be found. Every-thing follows from the creation of a limited number of Souls which gradually achieve purification and reunion with other purified Souls. The Zohar, a Kabalistic classic, believed to date back to the first century A.D., states:

   "The Souls must re-enter the Absolute whence they have emerged. But to accomplish this end, they must develop all the perfections, the germ of which is planted in them; and if they have not fulfilled this condition during one life, they must commence another, a third and so forth until they have acquired the condition which fits them for reunion with God."

   — The Case for Reincarnation (Page 90): Joe Fisher

Islam

10. "Transmigration or Tanasukh is viewed as inconsistent with the teachings of Prophet Mohammed, but the Quran says, quite explicitly":

    And Allah hath caused you to spring forth
    From the earth like a plant;
    Hereafter will He turn you back into it
    Again, and will bring you forth anew – Sura 71:17-18

    — The Case for Reincarnation Pages 89-90: Joe Fisher

35

The Doctrine of *Moksha* (Liberation)

We will now discuss what is *Moksha*? How can it be attained? And whether *Moksha* is an eternal state or it has a time-span?

Moksha as the Summum Bonum of Life

The Vedas, the Upanishads, the Gita and other scriptures of the Hindus proclaim that there is a purpose in life for which Man takes birth. According to these scriptures, the aim/purpose of life is to attain *Moksha*. Our scriptures talk of) '*Purušãrtha Chatušthya*' (100) i.e., four values for which man makes endeavours. These are *Dharma*, *Artha*, *Kama* and *Moksha*, the last being the ultimate goal. *Dharma* is righteousness, following the moral code of conduct; *Artha* is wealth and material gains; *Kama* is desires and longings for enjoyment and accomplishments; and *Moksha* is overcoming the Cycle of Birth and Death. The Vedic culture provides composite and wholesome life-style for all human beings. They are to earn wealth, enjoy life, but within the four walls of *Dharma* and thereafter attain *Moksha*.

The word *Moksha* means Liberation/Salvation/Enlightenment. Swami Dayanand was asked: What is *Moksha* (Liberation)? He replied that Liberation is that from which the people want to be liberated. From what the people want to be liberated? From sufferings. So, *Moksha* is to be liberated from sufferings. *Sankhya Darshana's* opening aphorism is:) ATHA TRIVIDHA DUKHÃTYANT NIVRITTIR ATYANTA PURUŠÃRTHAH, (101) i.e., we now propound the discipline of complete cesesion of three types of sufferings – *Adhyatmika* (Bodily), *Adhidaivika* (Natural Forces – like earthquake, flood, etc.) and *Adhibhautika* (from other beings, e.g., snake-bite or sufferings caused by fellow beings). That is why, while praying for peace, the word 'Shanti' is repeated thrice. Incidentally, Sigmund Freud also believes in three types of sufferings: "We are threatened with suffering from three directions: from our own body which is doomed to decay and destruction, from the external world – the merciless forces of destruction and finally from our relations to other men." In short, getting complete freedom from sufferings is *Moksha*.

Now, Soul can experience pleasure and pain only when in a body, a product of *Prakriti*. So, detachment of Soul from *Prakriti* is the sine qua non. When a Soul gets detached from *Prakriti* (*Prakriti Vimukta*), it resides in its own composed self. This is called state of *Kaivalya* or Self-Realisation. When Soul realises itself, God being Omnipresent resides in the Soul as well. So, the self-realisation is also god-realisation and that is *Moksha*. As God is all bliss (*Sachidananda*), Soul in God's lap attains a blissful state and becomes *Brahma-Rupa* (God-Like). Though the realised Soul does not become God or merge in God, it becomes god-like, blissful. A Sufi Persian poet has rightly said:

KHÃSÃNE KHUDÃ KHUDÃ NA BÃSHAND
ZE KHUDÃ JUDÃ NA BÃSHAND

i.e., the realised Souls do not become God, they are, verily, not separate from God. So, *Moksha* is the ultimate goal of Soul in taking birth. Same sentiment has been expressed by St. Thomas Aquinas: "Contemplation and vision of God is Man's absolute good."

Plato also describes how and when a Soul can reach the Abode of God:

"If the Soul takes its departure in a state of purity, not carrying with it any clinging impurities which during life, it never willingly shared in, but always avoided, gathering itself into itself and making this separation from the body its aim and study, well then, so prepared the Soul departs to that invisible region of the Divine, the Immortal, and the Wise."

What are the Means to Attain *Moksha*?

Before exploring the means, we may first analyse what is the cause of sufferings. The cause of sufferings of the Soul is its attachment with *Prakriti*. Yoga *Darshana* says: DRAŠTRI-DRISHYAYOH SANYOGO HEYAHETUH (102), i.e., the Union of the Seer (Soul) and the Seen (*Prakriti*) is the cause of sufferings. The blurring of the distinction between the Self and the *Prakriti* is due to *Avidya*. Strictly speaking, Soul's craving is for *Ananda*, Bliss, the source of which is God. But due to *Avidya* or *ignorance*, we get enamoured by the glamorous phenomenon of *Prakriti* and get engrossed in the sensory pleasures. And in pursuits of those pleasures, deny others their rightful dues and place and commit other heinous sins. We become self-centred and the Divine Spark in us becomes muddied. And all this we have been doing in life after life. So, the laws of *Karma*, as explained earlier, are operative in full force. The words of Dong Horton are relevant and helpful in this context. "We are all serving a life sentence, and good behaviour is our only hope for a pardon."

Nyaya Darshana (1.1.21-22) describes sufferings as: BÃDHANÃ LAKŠÑAM DUKHAM, TAḌATYANTA VIMOKŠO APAVARGAH (103), i.e., dependence or obstruction in fulfilling one's desires is the cause of sufferings. Complete annihilation of that is *Moksha*. That can be done by minimising our desires and that is possible by right type of knowledge. Right knowledge enables us to resist from bad deeds and inculcate in us the propensity to do good deeds. The cause of our birth, death and birth again is our sinful deeds and the only way to escape is good deeds and that is *Moksha*.

In this context, the prescription of the Vedas, Upanishads and the Gita is worthy of attention and practice:

ÎSHÃ-VÃSYAM-IDAM-SARVAM
YATKINCHIT JAGATYÃM JAGAT
TENA TAYAKTENA BHUNJÎTHÃ
MÃ GRIDDHAH KASYASVID-DHANAM (104)
(Yajur Veda – 40.8/Ishopanishad: Mantra 1)

i.e., all this, whatever moves in this moving world is pervaded with God. Therefore, enjoy the objects of nature with detachment. Do not covet others' wealth or do not covet, whom does this wealth belong? Nobody; it belongs to God. Dr. S. Radhakrishnan says "Sometimes this passage is interpreted as meaning: Enjoy what is allotted to you by God (Tena). Do not ask for more than what is given." "KASYASVID DHANAM, i.e., indeed whose wealth is it? It belongs to the Lord." Mahatma Gandhi says, "This *Mantra* tells me that I cannot hold as mine anything that belongs to God and that if my life... has to be a life of perfect dedication, it follows that it will have to be a life of continued service of fellow creatures." (Harijan 1937).

The next mantra of the Yajur Veda and Ishopanishad shows the way to liberation (*Moksha*):

KURVANNEVEHA KARMÃÑI
JIJÎVIŠET SHATAM SAMÃH
EVAM TAVAYI NÃNYATHETO ASTI
NA KARMA LIPYATE NARE (105)

i.e., while doing the deeds thus (without attachment), desire to live a hundred years. By so doing, Man is not bound by his *Karmas*. There is no other way.

This is the Gita's message of *Nishkam-Karma*. One has to do the *Karma*, but without attachment to its reward for Self. It contains a highly psychological truth. If one gets attached to his *Karma's* reward, he falls in the trap of doing wrong, undesirable deeds, because his intention is to get the reward by hook or by crook. The Gita and the Ishopanishad say perform the *Karmas* as a religious duty to serve the humanity. The Gita's Prescription (3.9) and *Nishkam Karma* is as follows:

YAJNÃRTHÃT KARMAÑO ANYATRA
LOKO AYAM KARMA-BANDHANAH
TADARTHAM KARMA KAUNTEYA
MUKTA SANGAH SAMÃCHAR (106)

i.e., in this world, any work, other than the one done with the intention of *Yajna* (service of others), is a cause of bondage. So, O Arjuna!, Act in that way and do that without any attachment, reward for self. The Soul of *Yajna* is IDANNA MAMA, i.e., this is not mine.

The Veda says 'RISHIH SA YO MANUR-HITAH' (107), i.e., he is a sage who is concerned with the interest of humanity. Aspirants of Yoga who dedicate their lives to service of humanity, without any desire for personal rewards attain *Moksha*. *Nishkama Karma* does not mean that it does not bring any reward to you. It only means you leave it to God. *Moksha*, in fact, is the reward of *Nishkama Karma*.

On Enlightenment

"It is the soul that is moved and awakened,
It is as if God drew back some of the many
Veils and coverings that are before it,
So that it might see what He is"

—John Yepes on Christ's Enlightenment

36
Is *Moksha* an Eternal State?

This is an established principle that whatever has a beginning must have an end. A Yogi after rigorous Yoga *Sadhna* or following rigorous moral, ethical, spiritual discipline and tirelessly working for the service of humanity in innumerable Cycles of Birth and Death and after God's grace attains *Moksha* at a point of time. Logically, the *Moksha* time-span must come to an end at some other point of time, howsoever inconceivably long that period may be.

In the Vedas, the Upanishads, the Gita and the *Darshanas*, cesesion of the Cycle of Birth and Death is called Moksha.

The Gita says:YAD GATVA NA NIVARTANTE TAD DHÃM PARAMAM MAMA (99), i.e., Having reached where they do not come back in this world, that is my Eternal Home. *Vedanta Darshana* (*Brahama Sutra*) says: ANÃVRITTI SHABDÃT (108), i.e., According to the Vedas, there is no return. *Sankhya Darshana* says: NA MUKTASYA PUNAR-BANDHA-YOGOAPI ANÃVRITTI SHRUTEH (109), i.e., the Released-Soul (Mukta-Atma) is not subject to the Cycle of Birth and Death as per the scriptures. These are all categorical and unambiguous statements that there is no return from the state of *Moksha*.

Adi Shankaracharya, Swami Dayanand Saraswati, Mundakopanishad and the *Sankhya Darshana* clarify this riddle. Adi Shankaracharya while commenting on the Chhandogya Upanishad's (8.15.1) declaration: NA CHA PUNARÃVARTANTE (110) i.e. And does not come back, says:

YÃVAT BRAHMALOKA STHITI TÃVAT TATRA EVA TIŠTHATI PRÃKTATO NÃVARTAT ITYARTHAH (111), i.e., it means that *Mukta-Jiva* stays in the *Brahma Loka* up to the allotted time and does not return prior to that. Swami Dayanand also interprets that the *Mukta Jiva* does not return to the world in ordinary sense of the word as we common beings do. They return after the specified period of *Mukti-Kãla* and he quotes the Mundukopanishad's Verse (3.2.6): TE BRAHRAM LOKE HA PRÃNTAKÃLE PARÃMRITÃT PARIMUCHANTI SARVE (112), i.e., they having stayed in Brahma Loka – enjoyed the bliss in the lap of God – leave that blissful state at the end of the great eon – *Prãntakãla*. Swami Dayanand calculates the *Prãntakãla*, on the basis of the shastras, as the period of 36,000 cycles of creation and dissolution (4.32 billion years × 2 × 36,000) which in human years comes to three hundred eleven trillion and forty billion years. This being so vast an expanse of time, we can legitimately say that they do not return to the world in the normal sense of the word.

For argument sake, if we presume that only one Soul attains *Moksha* in one cycle of creation and dissolution and does not return at all, then at some inconceivable remote time, all Souls will rest in God for all times to come and that as none will return, there will be an end to the cycle of creation and dissolution leaving God without His noble task of creation. *Sankhya Darshana* (1.159) assures us: IDÃNÎMIVA SARVATRA NA ATYANT-OCHHEDAH (113), i.e., This (Cycle of Creation and Dissolution) is eternal, there is no complete cessation of it.

Now the question arises why there is widespread belief that the *Mukta Jiva* does not return from the state of *Moksha* despite the aforesaid scriptural references as also the following categorical declaration of the Gita (9.21):

TE TAM BHUKTVÃ SVARGA LOKAM VISHÃLAM

KŠÎÑE PUÑYE MARTYA-LOKAM VISHANTI (114), i.e., they after enjoying the bliss in the great paradise return to this mortal world on the exhaustion of their good deeds' fruit.

The persistence in the belief in non-return from *Moksha* is partly due to lack of study, not going beyond the literal meaning of NA NIVARTANTE, i.e., they do not return. It is also largely due to the spiritual blindness of some devotees who believe Svarga (Paradise) is different from *Brahma Loka* (Abode of God). They believe that the *Mukta Jivas* reside in God eternally, but somewhat other noble Souls, who have not yet attained *Moksha*, reside in *Svarga*, enjoy and come back. In fact, in the Vedic lexion *Moksha*, *Param Dham*, *Param Gati*,

Svarga are synonyms. They all mean to reside in God and not in some fanciful place called *Svarga*. The Shiv Gita clarifies: MOKŠASYA NAHI VÃSOASTI GRÃMVISHEŠAH (115), i.e., *Moksha* is not some specified place where *Mukta Atmas* reside in God.

To sum up, the *Moksha* is not eternal. It is time-bound. The *Mukta-Jivas* return and the bound *Jivas* attain *Moksha* and enjoy the bliss in the lap of God and this cycle goes on perenially. Its further corollary is that we all have enjoyed the *Moksha* bliss in the past and will enjoy it again at some remote point of time.

Dedication to God

"To do the will of God: the exterior will,
the interior will, the essential will.
To do it for the sake of God alone, and without reference to what he himself desired, or hoped, or might gain in this world or the next .... To annihilate himself in all he thought and felt and did, so that there should be nothing left but the instrument of God's will and a soul united by God's grace with that divine substance, which was identical with the divine, essential will."

—Aldous Huxley

37
Belief in Return from Liberated State (*Moksha*) in Non-Hindu Cultures

Incidentally, apart from the Hindus, the ancient Egyptian and the Hebrew civilisations also believed not only in the concept of *Moksha*, but also in the return to the world after enjoying the company of God. The following passages are worthy of attention:

"The ancient Egyptians spoke of sensitive Souls passing through the gate of Gods into AMENTHE (Paradise) where they dwelt in continuous bliss, until descending once more to animate a new body."

— Joe Fisher: The Case for Reincarnation (Pages 120-121)

"Similarly, the Hebrews of old envisaged a spell in PARDISH or Paradise ... Souls whose time in Pardish has nearly expired are given instructions for the next life, explains the ZOHAR (Hebrew Scripture), before being sent out 'sorrowing in exile'; to a place where there is no true happiness because only in the presence of God can this state be attained."

— Joe Fisher: The Case for Reincarnation (Page 121)

In Christianity too, we find references to God realisation, Salvation (*Moksha*), e.g.,

"And now, O Father, glorify Thou me with Thine own self,
with the glory which I had with Thee before the world was."

— The Holy Bible (John 17.5)

"Truly my soul waiteth upon God:
from Him cometh my salvation."

— The Holy Bible (Psalm 62.1)

38

Yoga – The Workshop of Indian Culture and Philosophy

The purpose of detailed discussion on the Fundamentals of Ancient Indian Philosophy is to make the Yoga aspirants aware of the whole gamut of Sage Patanjali's philosophy on which his Yoga *Darshana* is based and about which the Sage himself does not proffer any details. He presumes that the Yoga aspirant is aware of what forms the matrix of Indian philosophy and culture and proceeds to propound his system of Yoga. Dr. Radhakrishan has succinctly observed in his book 'Indian Philosophy', "The main interest of Patanjali is not metaphysical theorising, but the practical motive of indicating how salvation can be attained by disciplined activities."

To elucidate this point, given below are Saga Patanjali's presumptions: When he advises *Chiita-Vritti Nirodha* in the very second *Sutra* of his treatise, the existence of Soul who is to do it, is accepted as an undisputed fact. When the Sage prescribes *Ishvara-Pranidhana* as an aid to *Samadhi*, existence of God is presumed. When the Sage states) BHOG-APVARGARTHAM DRISHYM, (70) i.e., the created world is for the enjoyment and Liberation of Soul, the existence of *Prakriti* is taken for granted. When the Sage says: SATI MÛLE TADVIPÃKO JÃTYRÃYUR BHOGAH (116) Yoga Darshana (II.13), i.e., with the existence of cause (*Karma* and *Avidya*), the result is acquiring a life-form, life-span and experiencing pleasure and pain, the Sage's belief in the Doctrine of *Karma* and the Doctrine of Reincarnation stands established. And, finally, when he talks of *Kaivalya*, his belief in *Moksha* is also proved. In short, Sage Patanjali does not feel the necessity of explaining the concepts which are well proved and well accepted in Vedas, the Upanishads and other Shastras and straightaway proceeds with his subject-matter. That is why, the Yoga *Darshana* is very crisp, the shortest among the six *Darshanas* and the most effective and practical – a handbook to the gateway of *Moksha*.

Yoga is the workshop of Indian culture and philosophy. While the *Brahma-Sutra* (*Vedanta Darshana*) satisfies our curiosity about God, Yoga *Darshana* makes us see God. Through the prescription of *Yama* and *Niyama*, it chastens our Souls, makes us shed the dross that envelops us. Through the *Asana*, *Pranayama* and *Pratyahara*, it prepares our mind for concentration. And through *Dhãrãna*, *Dhyãn* and *Samadhi*, it opens new vistas of our mind, and elevates our Soul to gain supernatural powers and ultimately leads us to realise ourselves as to who we are and for what purpose we have come in this world. And when the Soul is seated in its original unperturbed, composed state, it sees God and rests in Him.

Thus Spake Scholars on Vedas

"The Vedas, I feel convinced will occupy scholars for centuries to come, and we take and maintain forever its position as the most ancient of books in the library of mankind."

—Prof. F. Max Muller
India : What Can It Teach Us?

"Whenever I have read any part of the Vedas, I have felt that some unearthly unknown light illuminated me."

—Henry David Thoreau

39
Arise! Awake!

It is fortunate that we are born in India and have imbibed the eternal Indian Culture with the milk of our mother's breast. It is our bounden duty to preserve and practise the values enshrined in the culture and imbue the same in our children lest they get swept off their feet by the wave of materialism and the gale of sensuous propaganda of the Western culture of 'eat, drink and be merry'. Maharishi Aurobindo has observed "Bharat is *Karma-Bhumi*, other countries are *Bhog-Yoni.*" The same sentiment is expressed by Omar Ben Hashaam, the uncle of Prophet Mohammed.

"O God! Take away my whole life and grant me only one day's stay in India because having reached there, man attains liberation."

— (Se Arul Okool Page 235)

The Upanishadic clarion call is: UTTIŠTHATA JÃGRATA PRÃPYA VARÃN NIBODHAT (117), i.e., Arise! Awake! Approach the noble and gain wisdom, acquaint and fortify yourself with the time-tested values of your culture; Try to know: What is the purpose of life; What are your duties regarding yourself, your family, your society, your nation and the world. Perform those duties with dedication, and you will have peace, joy, respect, progress and satisfaction in life.

We can ignore the said call of the Upanishad at our own peril as advised by John Milton in Paradise Lost, "Arise, Awake, or be forever fallen." Mohammed Iqbal's words also serve as a warning: VATAN KÎ FIKR KAR NÃDÃN MUSÎBAT ÃNE WÃLI HAI, i.e., O Ignorant one! Worry about the nation, trouble is in the offing.

Ours is a well-respected, well-admired culture, the matrix of which is spirituality. The following words of renowned philosophers indicate what India is and what it stands for:

"India is the cradle of the human race, the birthplace of human speech, the mother of history, the grandmother of legend and the great grandmother of tradition."

—Mark Twain

"India will teach us the tolerance of the mature mind, the quiet content of the unacquisitive Soul, the calm of the understanding spirit, and a unifying, purifying love for all living things."

—Will Durant (Our Oriental Heritage)

Our Civilisation and culture have survived the vicissitudes of time, the onslaught of foreign invasions and the subjugation during foreign rule only because of its spiritual content. Swami Vivekananda reminds us, "Spider weaves the web where Caesar ruled." Similarly, the Egyptian civilisation of time-defying Pyramids and well-preserved thousands of years' old Mummies is extinct. As against this, our culture and civilisation are intact. The values for which India is known are still prevalent in its people earning the epithet, 'Every Indian is a born philosopher'. These values can be seen in the towering personalities of Mahatma Buddha, Adi Shankaracharya, Guru Nanak, Swami Dayananda, Swami Vivekananda, Aurobindo Ghosh and Mahatma Gandhi who by their living examples demonstrated that the values of Ahimsa, Truth, Compassion, Control over one's senses, Renunciation, Service of Humanity are not only to be read in scriptures or history books, but these are to be practised in life.

Swami Vivekananda assures us with a caution, "The Indian Nation cannot be killed. Deathless it stands and it will stand so long as that spirit shall remain as the background; so long as her people do not give up their spirituality."

That spirit of India is reflected in the *Yogic* and *Yâjnic* (pronounced as *Yâgyic*) attitude of its people. The spirit of Yoga is for individual's personal spiritual elevation and the spirit of *Yajna* (*Yagya*) for the well-being of society. The Soul of *Yajna* is: IDANNA MAMA, i.e., this is not mine. All wealth has been bestowed on us by God and, therefore, while using it with detachment, it is to be spent for the well-being of humanity. *Yajna* is not *Agnihotra* (Oblation to Fire) alone, any act of well being of others is *Yajna*.

Defining 'Virtue' and 'Sin', a poet has said:

AŠTÃDASHA PURÃÑEŠÛ
VYÃSASYA VACHANAM DVAYAM

PROPAKÃRH PUÑYÃYA
PÃPÃYA PARA PÎRNAM (118)

i.e., in 18 Puranas, Sage Vyasa has stated two things: Well-being of others is 'Virtue' and hurting others is 'Sin'.

The philosophy and practice of Yoga is essential not only for spiritual elevation of our individual beings, but is also equally, in fact more essential for administrators, rulers , military personnel, world leaders, and dictators because on their actions, good, bad are wrong, depends the destiny of millions of people.

India's great political thinker Acharya Chanakya has stated: SUKHASYA MÛLAM DHARMAM, DHARMASYA MÛLAM ARTHAM, ARTHASYA MÛLAM RAJYAM (149). i.e. Source of Happiness is Dharma – Righteousness ; Source of Righteousness is Artha – Wealth – all activities of well being of others require wealth and Source of Artha is Rajyam – The State i.e well governance. If there is no law and order, there is no just system of dispensation of justice, no recognition of merit ; if officials and rulers are corrupt and nepotists, there cannot be peace, prosperity and happiness among the people in the state.

It is, therefore, incumbent that administrators and rulers with onerous responsibilities of State, have calm, composed and ethical attitude in their functioning. They have to rise above self-interest (Nija-hita) and work in public interest (Jan-hita) and national interest (Rashtra-hita). But even the national interest has to be circumscribed by the interest of humanity at large.

The world today is perched on a mountain of nuclear weapons and any misadventure on the part of some egocentric rulers may result in annihilation of human existence on earth. The Yogic prescriptions will curb their senseless rivalries, overweening ambitions, calm down their surcharged tempers and make them behave sanely. The Atharva Veda's dictum (12.1.12) in this context will serve as panacea:

MÃTÃ BHŨMI PUTRO AHAM PRITHIVYÃH (150)
(The country of my birth is my Mother;
I am the Son of the planet Earth.)

Meaning thereby, while pursuing the national interest of one's own country, one should not subjugate others' countries or plunder earth's resources or threaten its existence, because one's own country is only a limb of Mother Earth and one should protect the whole earth as a dutiful Son. That is why our scriptures declare VASUDHAIVA

KUTUMBKAM (13) i.e. the whole world is a family. That is why H.G. Wells stated: 'Our true nationality is Mankind'. Realizing the gravity of wars and ethnic conflicts, French philosopher Romain Rolland stated: "Yoga is the gift of the ancient times, even of unearthly civilization and if we do not use the knowledge of millennia, we will lose one of the chances for survival". American philosopher Mark Twain expressed the same sentiment: "At this extremely dangerous moment in human history the only way of salvation is the ancient Hindu way."

Now that the United Nations has recognized the universal appeal of Yoga and declared 21st June as International Day of Yoga, the leaders of the world should not treat it only as an Annual Physical Exercise Event, but imbibe the ethical and moral content of Yoga in their lives, to make this planet a paradise on earth.

Conclusion

We have described in this book the philosophy of Yoga as also the ancient Indian Philosophy on which the Yoga system is based. We will now impart lessons in practising Yoga. Just as for an experiment, theoretical knowledge of the object, on which experiment is to be conducted, is necessary, detailed background of ancient Indian Philosophy is necessary for proper understanding of the Yoga discipline. This will invoke in the aspirants due faith in the system and that will give him better results.

We can't make a tall claim that our preliminary lessons in practising Yoga will earn the readers the *Vibhuties* or *Siddhies* (Supernatural Powers) that advanced Yogis gain after rigorous Sadhana, or that any aspirant will attain *Moksha* which the Yogis attain after persistent *Sadhana* in innumerable lives (what the Gita calls *Aneka Janama Sansiddhi*).

All the same, we do earnestly hope if Yoga is practised in all its aspects – Moral Discipline, Physical exercises, Breathing Exercises and Meditation – this book will help the readers enlarge their consciousness and develop their personality to achieve good health, sharp memory, penetrating intellect, professional proficiencies, better interpersonal relationship, moral strength, and, above all, bring in inner peace and richness in their lives.

Section III

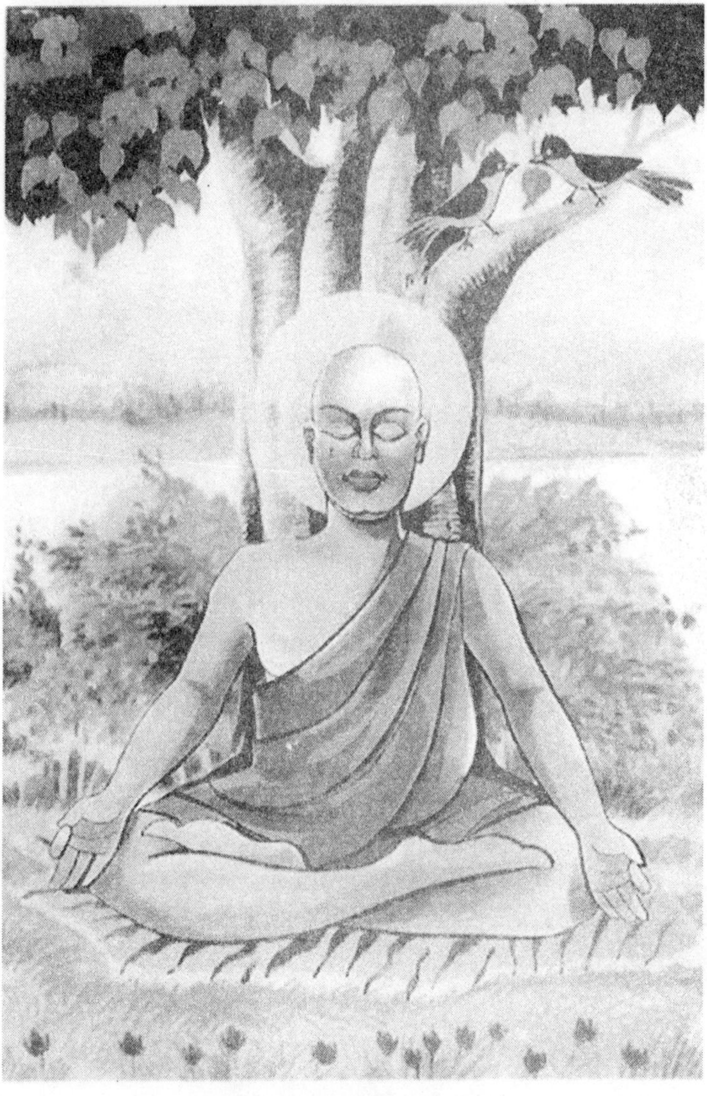

योगश्चित्तवृत्तिनिरोधः

चित्त की वृत्ति या कहो कि गतिविधि
पर, अंकुश लगाना है योग ।

Controlling the modifications of mind is Yoga

Vedic Nectar

YADAGNE SYÃM AHAM TVAM
TVAM VÃ YÃ SYÃ AHAM
SYUŠTE SATYÃ IH ÃSHIŠAH (119)

—Rig Veda 8.44.23

O divine Agni : Self Refulgent God !
If I become you
Or you become I
You will realise my difficulties
And shower your blessings
On me here and now.

40
Practical Lessons in Yoga

Sage Patanjali's *Ashtanga* Yoga – Eight-Part Yoga is meant for ordinary people who have no grounding or experience in Yoga. It is a system of educating, chiselling and elevating those people who pick up fights at the drop of a hat; do not hesitate to tell lies to grind their axe; are avaricious, lustful and self-centred, prone to evading government taxes and taking bribes; and having no compunctions in adulterating food-stuffs or medicines for their monetary gains. For these common individuals, Sage Patanjali opens the door for attaining blissful state.

Sage Patanjali imbues in them moral values through *Yama* and *Niyama*. Briefs them about their true identity – Immortal Souls, quite distinct from *Prakriti* which ensnares them with worldly attractions. Teaches them their goal in life – Self-Realisation, leading to God-Realisation and perennial Bliss.

God or Nature has blessed us with three organs – Head, Heart and Hand. Head is the representative of intellectual faculties; Heart is the representative of emotional makeup and Hand is the representative of will-power. In other words, Head represents Knowledge (Gyan), Heart represents Devotion (Bhakti) and Hand represents Action (Karma). For a balanced life, all the three must act in unison. Knowledge and Action without Devotion lead to selfishness, e.g., bridge falls before inauguration. Action and Devotion without true Knowledge can lead to blind faith and fanaticism. Knowledge and Devotion without Action sterile, of no use to society.

King Ravana was a great scholar. He is said to have written commentary on the Vedas, but he did not practise the teachings of the Vedas in his life. For such persons, Rig Veda says YASTANNA

VEDA KIMRICHÃ KRIŠYATI (120), i.e., who does not know Him what can the *Veda Mantra* do to him? Nothing. Dante has also said exactly the same thing, "What shall one do with the Verse if he knows not That." The same sentiment is expressed in the Welsh Proverb: "A spoon does not know the taste of soup, nor a learned fool the taste of wisdom."

For the true Yoga aspirants, Sage Patanjali has prescribed four qualifications or prerequisites: *Shradhã* (Faith in the Yoga System), *Vîrya* (Energy to undertake Relentless Efforts), *Smriti* (Constant Remembrance of the tenets of Yoga Discipline) and *Samadhi-Pragya* (Pure intellect to pursue *Samadhi*).

In short, mere intellectual knowledge about the Yoga philosophy is not adequate. It needs to be put to practice in life ardently and earnestly. That will chisel the Divine Spark in the aspirant and change his life forever. Shvetashvar Upanishad (2.12) says:

NA TASYA ROGO NA JARÃ NA MRITYUH
PRÃPTASYA YOGA-AGNIM AYAM SHRÎRAM (121),
(One whose body is castigated by the heat of Yoga
Suffers from neither Disease nor Oldage nor Death.)

Though the aforesaid is the highly advanced stage of Yoga Sadhana, not withstanding, the beginning can be made with short steps. Practical lessons in Yoga have been given in this section in four steps: Step I – Moral Discipline, Step II – Asana, Step III – Pranayama, Step IV– Meditation. Photographs of Postures of Yoga Asanas and Pranayama Kriyas have been given in the beginning of this section. The Yoga Practitioners are advised to refer to these while practising Yoga.

May God bless all aspirants!

Do you know what was The First ever Gramophone Recording!

When Thomas Edison invented the gramophone record, in 1877 which could record human voice for posterity, he wanted to record the voice of an eminent scholar Prof. F. Max Muller on his first piece. Accordingly, at the inaugural ceremony, Max Muller came on the stage and spoke in front of the instrument. Later the gramophone disc was played and the following was heard:

AGNI MÎLE PUROHITAM YAJNASYAS DEVAM RITVIJAM HOTÃRAM RATNADHÃTAMAM (151)

The audience was thrilled to hear the voice of Max Muller from the instrument. After several rounds of applause by the audience and congratulations to Thomas Alwa Edison, Max Muller came on the stage and addressed the scholars and asked them:

"You heard my original voice in the morning. Then you heard the same voice coming out from this instrument in the afternoon. Do you understand what I said in the morning or what you heard in the afternoon?".

The audience fell silent because they could not understand the language in which Max Muller had spoken. Max Muller then explained what he had spoken. He said that the language he spoke was Sanskrit and it was the first Mantra of Rig Veda. (1.1.1)

Why did Max Muller choose this? Addressing the audience he said, "Vedas are the oldest text of the human race. And Agni Meele Purohitam is the first verse of Rig Veda. In the most primordial time, when the people did not know how even to cover their bodies and lived by hunting and housed in caves, Indians had attained high civilisation and they gave the world universal philosophies in the form of the Vedas".

When "Agni Meele Purohitam" was replayed the entire audience stood up in silence as a mark of respect for the ancient Indian Sages. This verse means:

"Oh Agni,You who gleam in the darkness, to You we come day by day, with devotion and bearing homage. So be of easy access to us, Agni, as a father to his son, abide with us for our well being."

—(Source Internet)

In the Vedas, word Agni is used for God as well. Prof. Max Muller also has stated this. (See page 79) Taking the meaning of Agni as God, Swami Dayananda Sarasvati has interpreted this Mantra as follows:

O Effulgent God, the Provider of all knowledge the Benefactor, the Creator of the Universe and the Source of all wealth! I adore Thee.

—Author

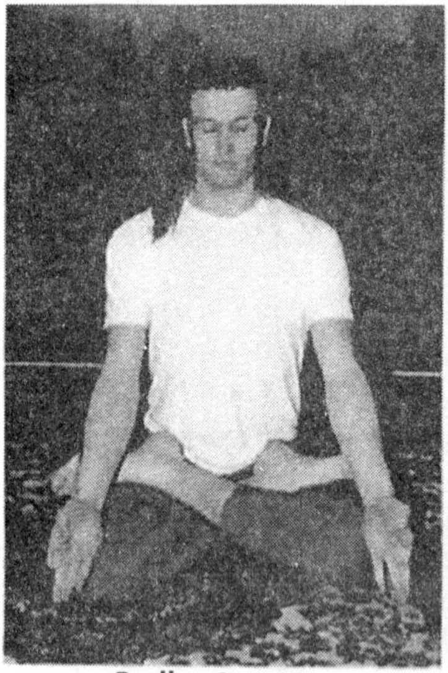

Padha Asana
(Mediative Posture)
पद्मासन (ध्यान मुद्रा)

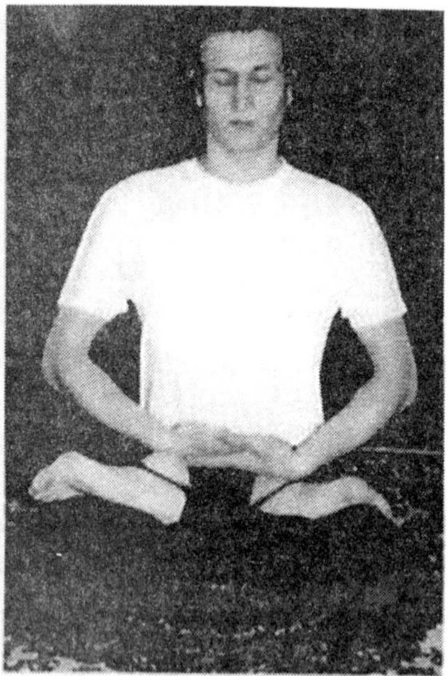

Padha Asana
(Swastika Posture)
पद्मासन (स्वस्तिका मुद्रा)

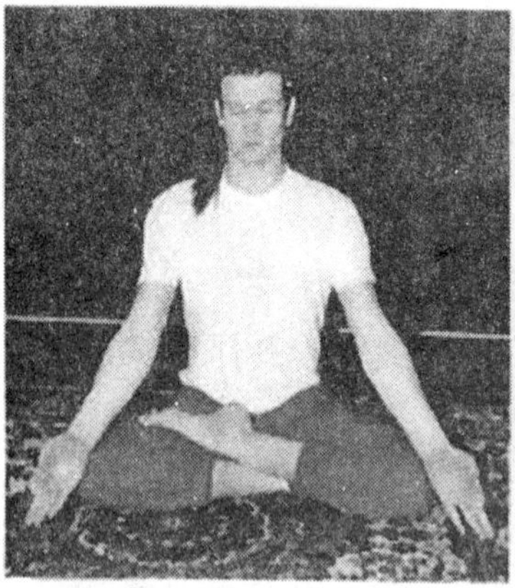

Ardha Padma Asana
(Half Lotus Posture)
अर्द्ध पद्मासन

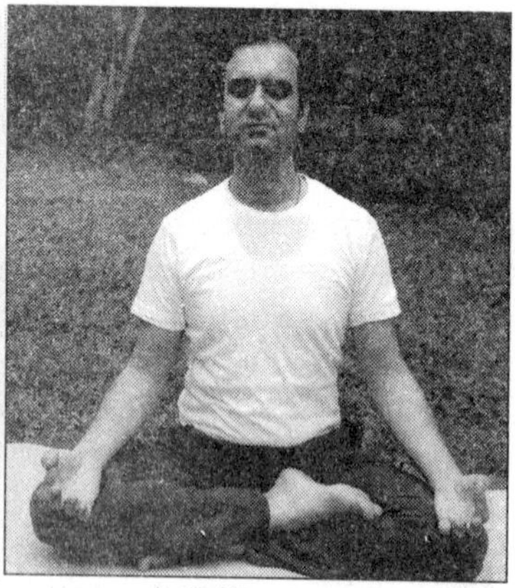

Sidha Asana
(Enligtened-Person Posture)
सिद्धासन

* शोधकर्ताओं का मत है कि पद्मासन सुखासन आदि पिरामिड △ का आकार होने के कारण अधिक शान्तिप्रद हैं।

Researches have found that Padma Asana, Sukh Asana etc. provide more peace and tranquility being in pyramid shape.

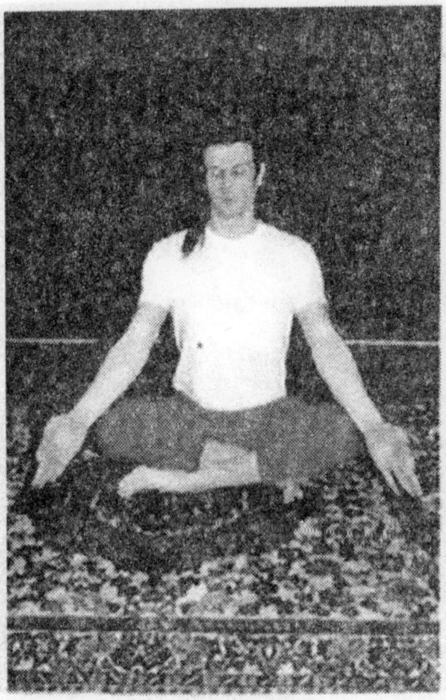

Sukh Asana
(Cross legged Posture)
सुखासन

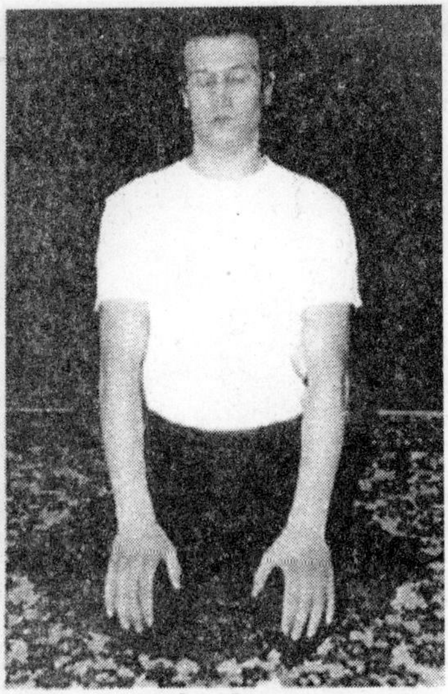

Vajra Asana
(Front Posture)
वज्रासन (सामने की स्थिति)

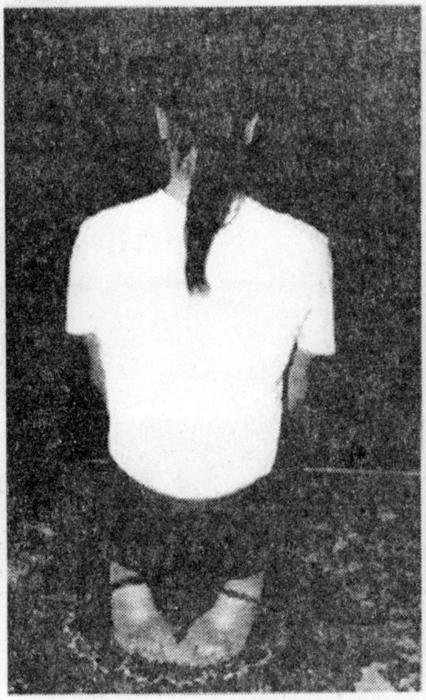

Vajra Asana
(Back Posture)
वज्रासन (पीछे की स्थिति)

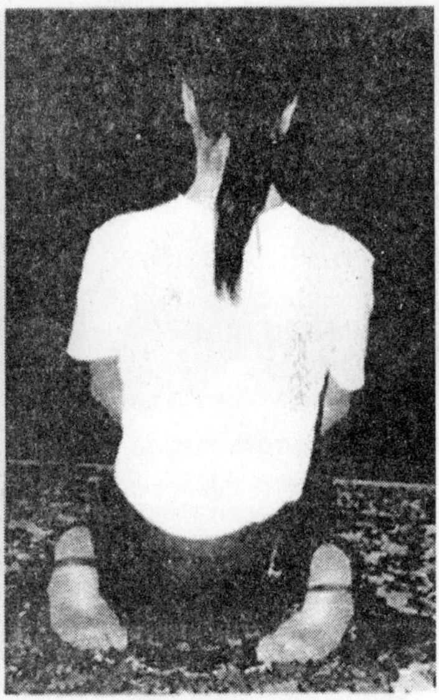

Vajra Asana
(Back Posture)
वज्रासन (पीछे की स्थिति)

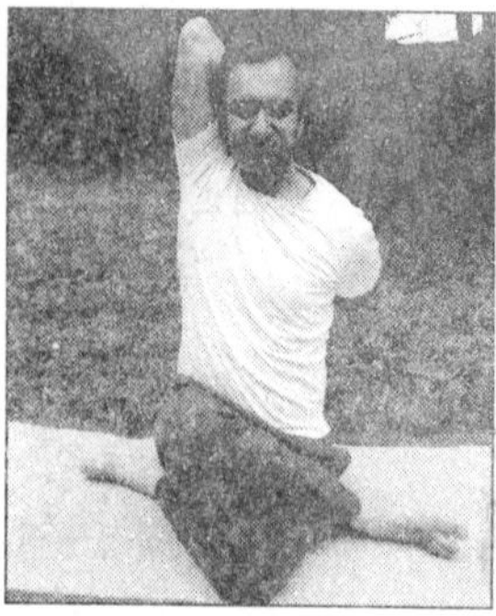

Gomukh Asana (Cow-Head Front Posture)

गोमुखासन

(सामने की स्थिति)

Gomukh Asana (Cow-Head Back Posture)

गोमुखासन

(पीछे की स्थिति,

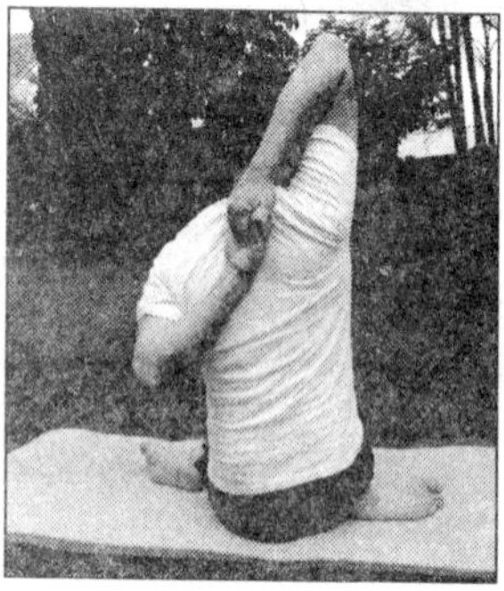

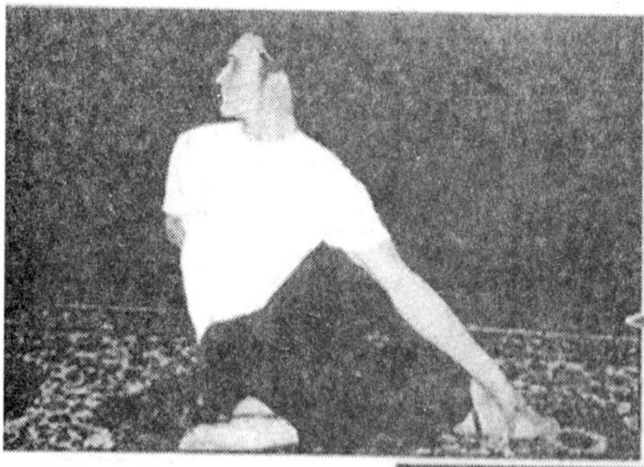

Ardhamatsyendra Asana (Spinal Twist Front Posture)

अर्द्धमत्स्येन्द्र आसन

(सामने की स्थिति)

Ardhamatsyendra Asana (Spinal Twist Back Posture)

अर्द्धमत्स्येन्द्र आसन

(पीछे की स्थिति)

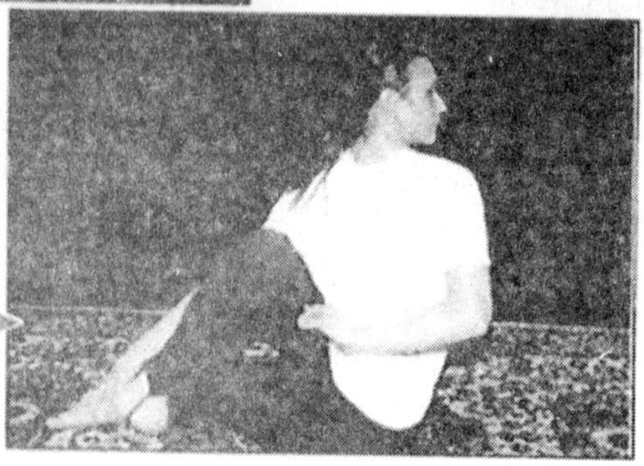

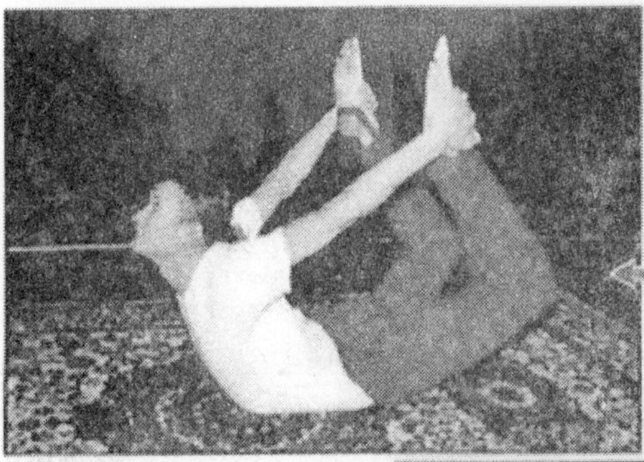

Dhanur Asana (Bow Posture)

धनुरासन

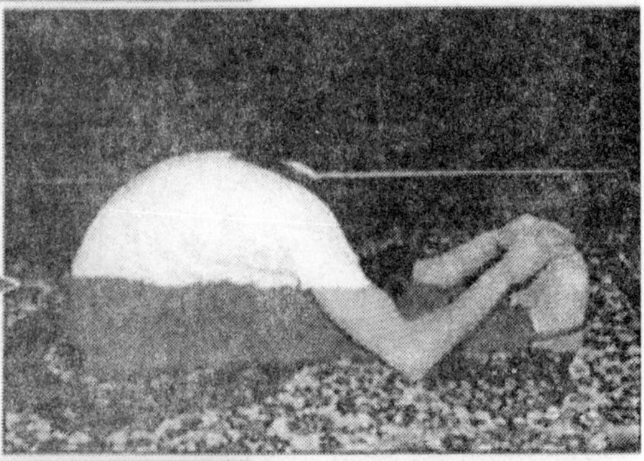

Pashchimotton Asana (Forward-Bending Posture)

पश्चिमोत्तान आसन

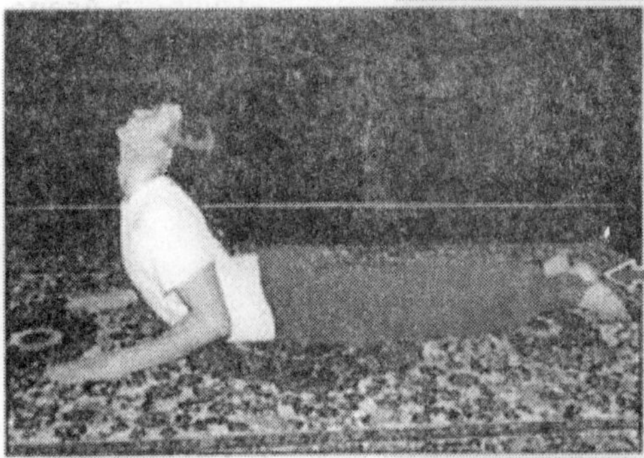

Bhujanga Asana (Cobra Posture)

भुजंगासन

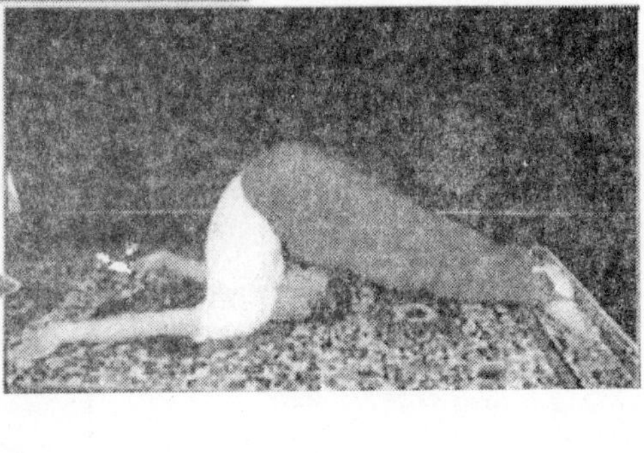

Hala Asana (Plough Posture)

हलासन

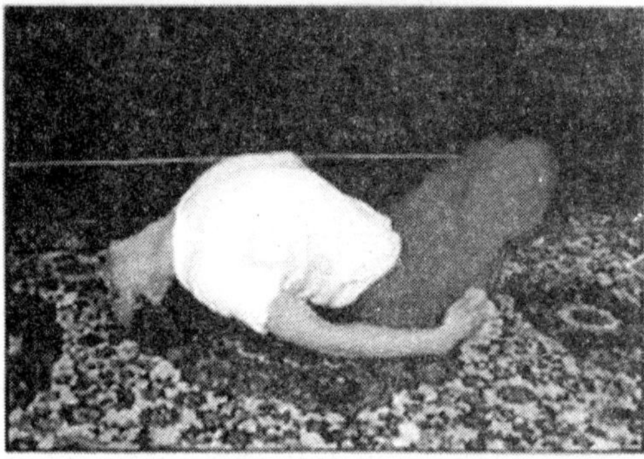

Matsya Asana
(Fish Posture)

मत्स्यासन

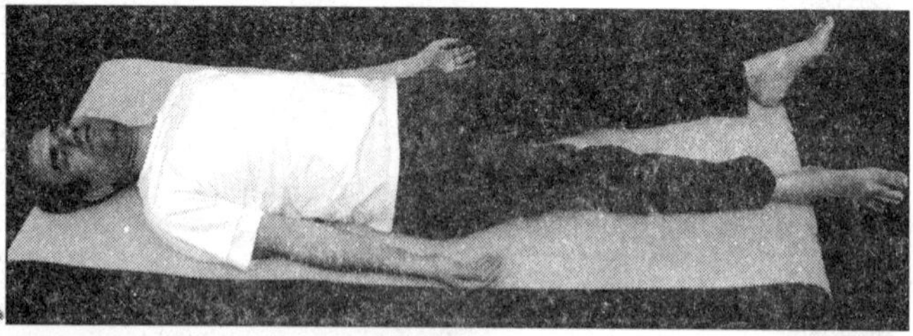

शवासन

Shava Asana
(Dead-body Posture)

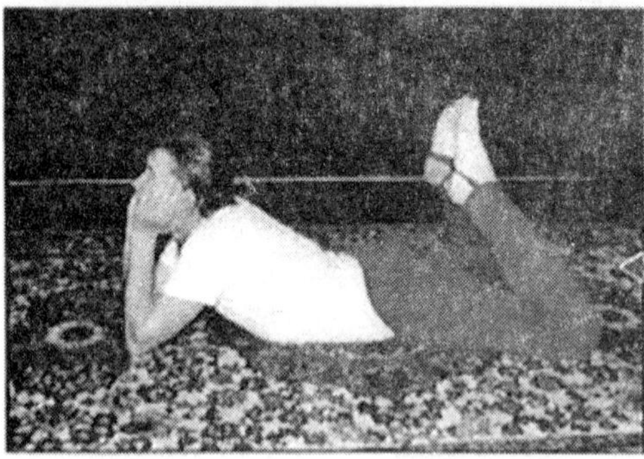

Makar Asana
(Crocodile Posture)

मकर आसन

Nadi Shodan
(Cleansing of Nerves)
Pranayama

नाड़ी शोधन

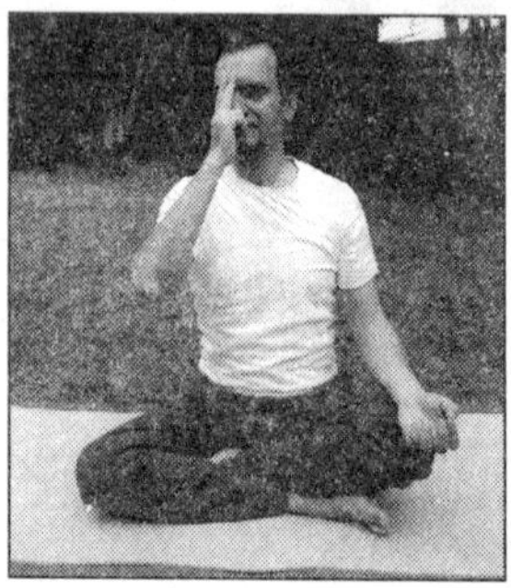

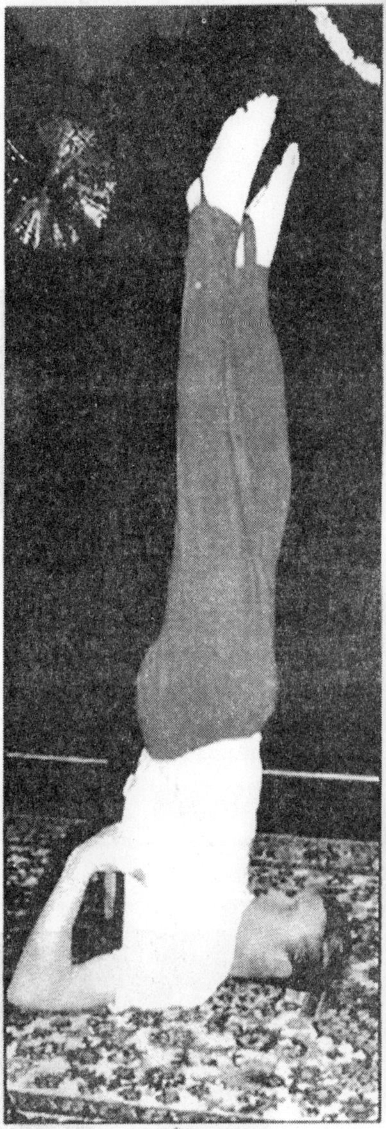

सर्वाङ्गासन

Sarvanga Asana (All-Limbs Posture)

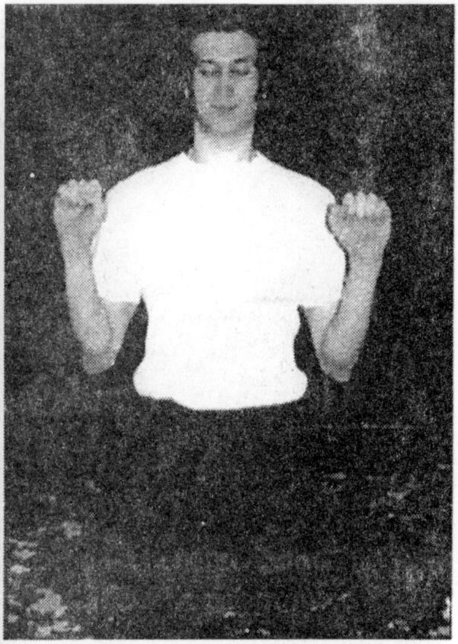

भस्त्रिका (पहली स्थिति)

Bhastrika (Bellow Breathing) First Posture

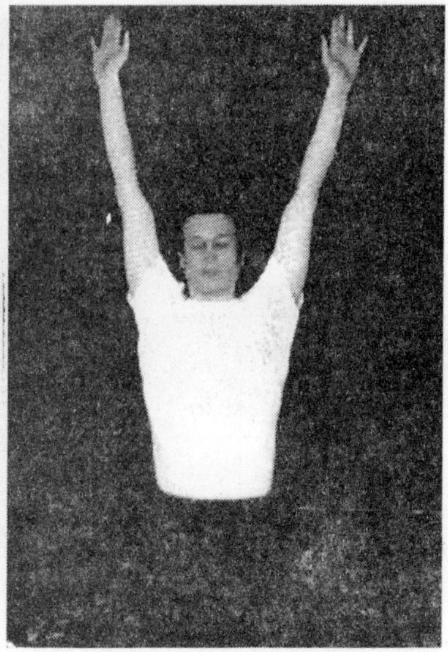

भस्त्रिका (दूसरी स्थिति)

Bhastrika (Bellow Breathing) Second Posture

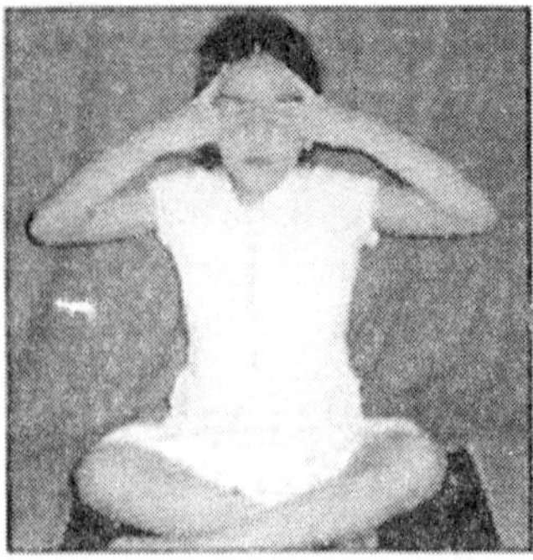

Bhramari (Bumble Bee) Pranayama

भ्रामरी

Three Stage Pranayama (Belly Posture: Inhalation)

त्रिदेशी (कटी मुद्रा) :
(पूरक स्थिति)

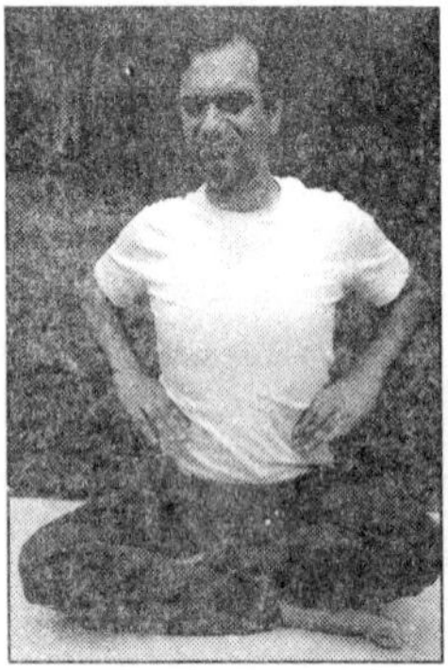

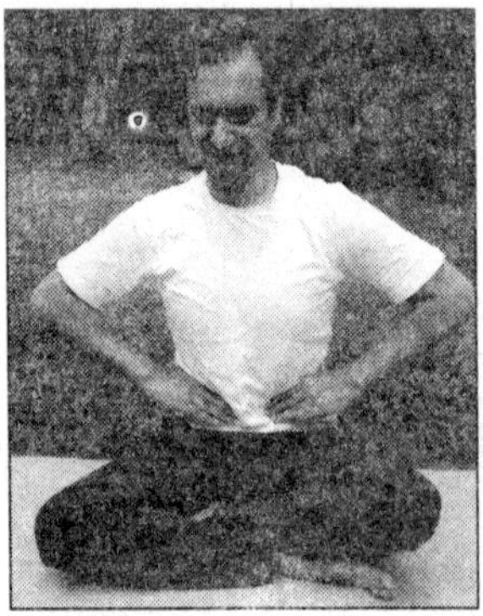

Three Stage Pranayama (Belly Posture: Exhalation)

त्रिदेशी (कटी मुद्रा) :
रेचक स्थिति

Three Stage Pranayama (Chest Posture: Inhalation)

त्रिदेशी (वक्ष: स्थल मुद्रा)
(पूरक स्थिति)

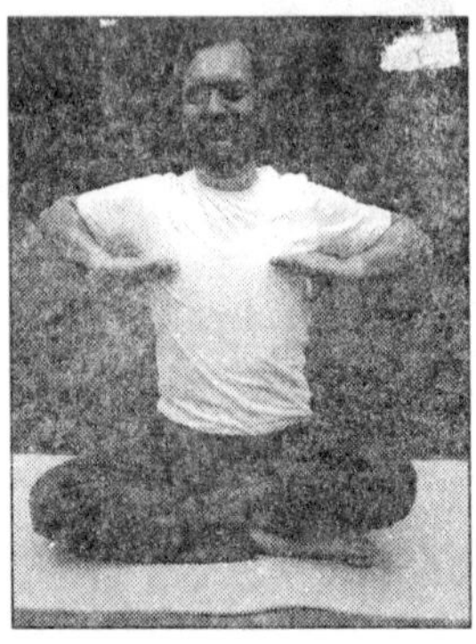

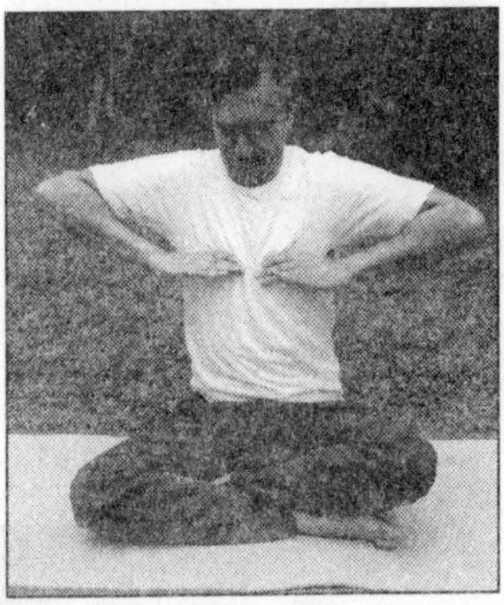

Three Stage Pranayama (Chest Posture: Exhalation)

त्रिदेशी (वक्ष:स्थल मुद्रा)
(रेचक स्थिति)

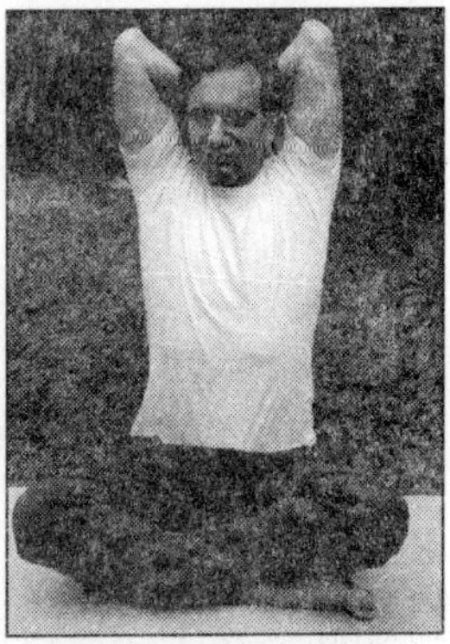

Three Stage Pranayama (Shoulder Posture)

त्रिदेशी (स्कन्ध मुद्रा)

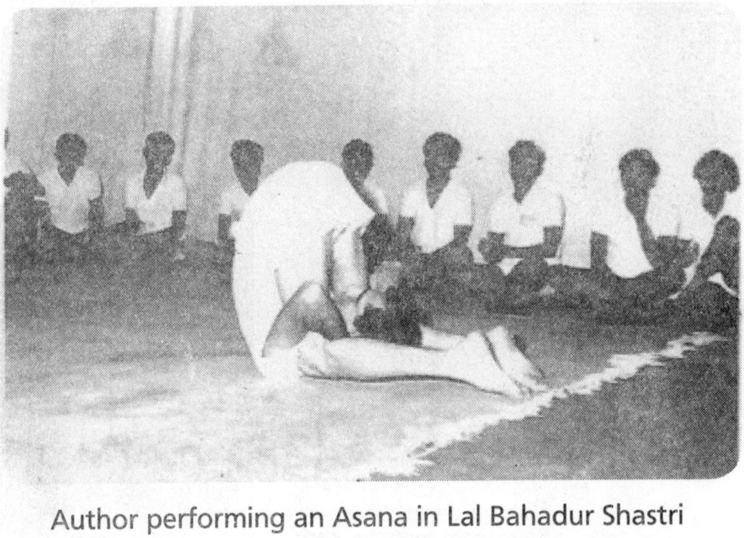

Author performing an Asana in Lal Bahadur Shastri Academy in Mussoorie in 1974 during training.

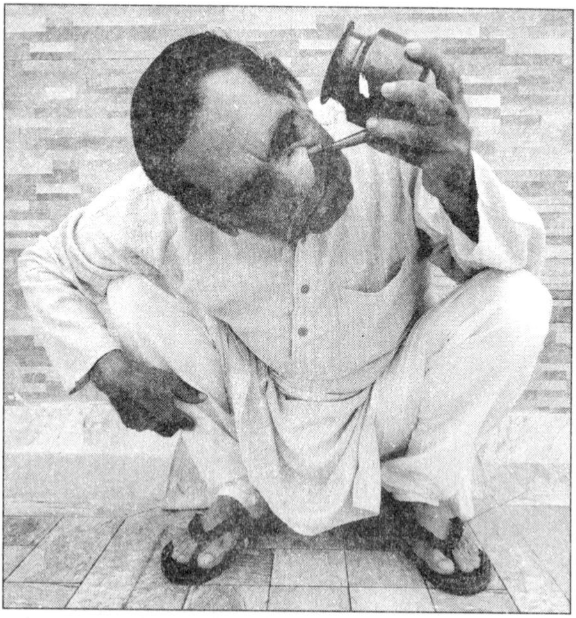

Nasal Cleansing जल नेति

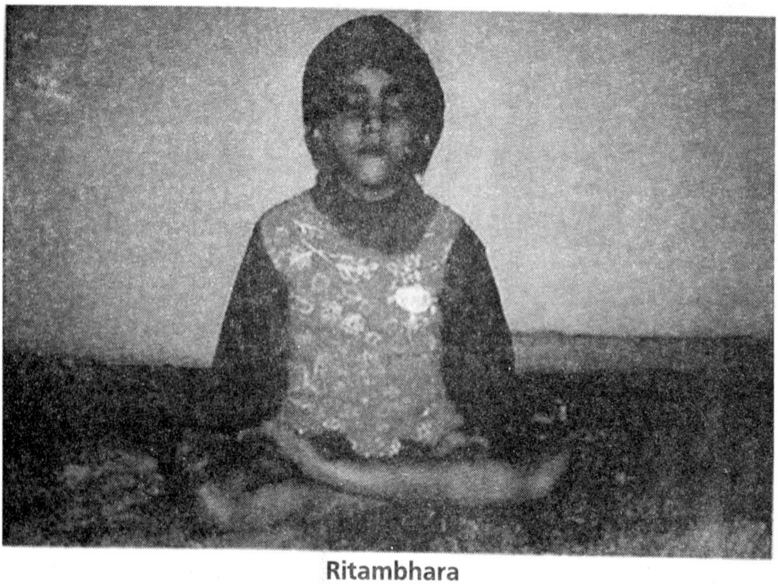

Ritambhara
(Grand-daughter of the Author)

ऋतम्भरा (लेखक की दौहित्री)

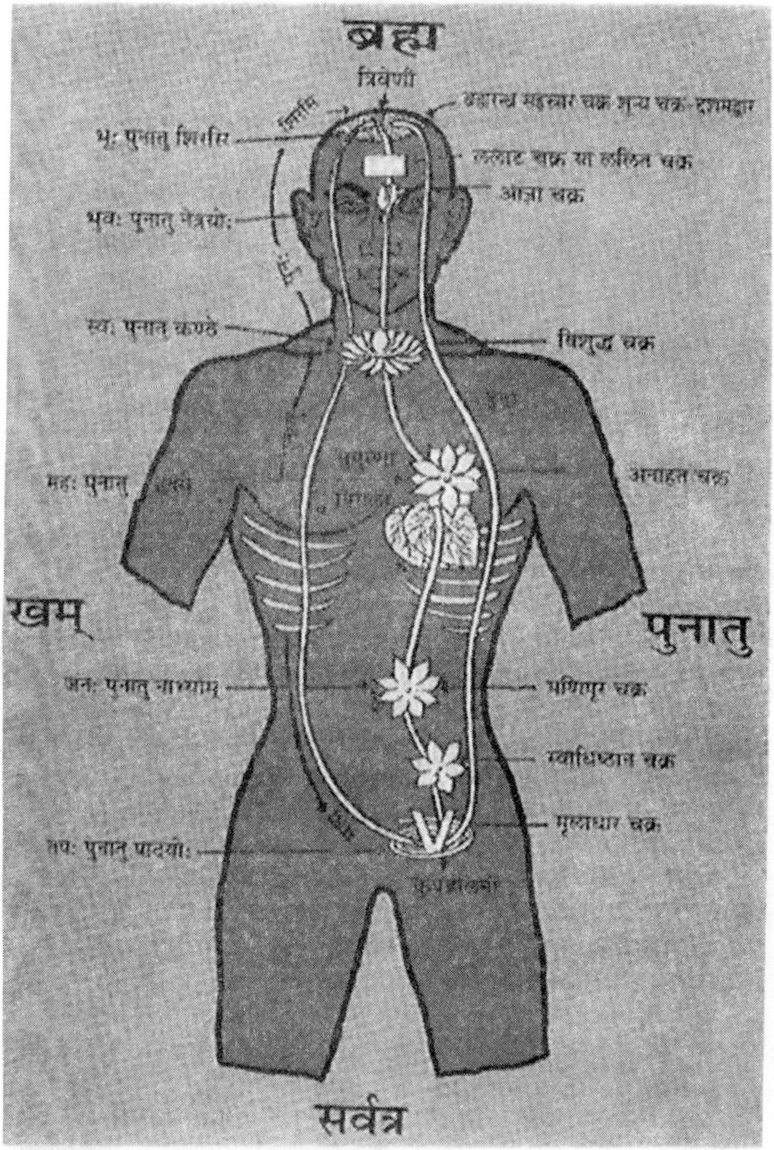

Eight Chakras अष्टचक्र

(आचार्य विश्वश्रवाकृत सन्ध्यापद्धतिमीमांसा से साभार उद्धृत)

(By courtesy- Archaya Vishvashrava'Sandhapathati-Mimansa)

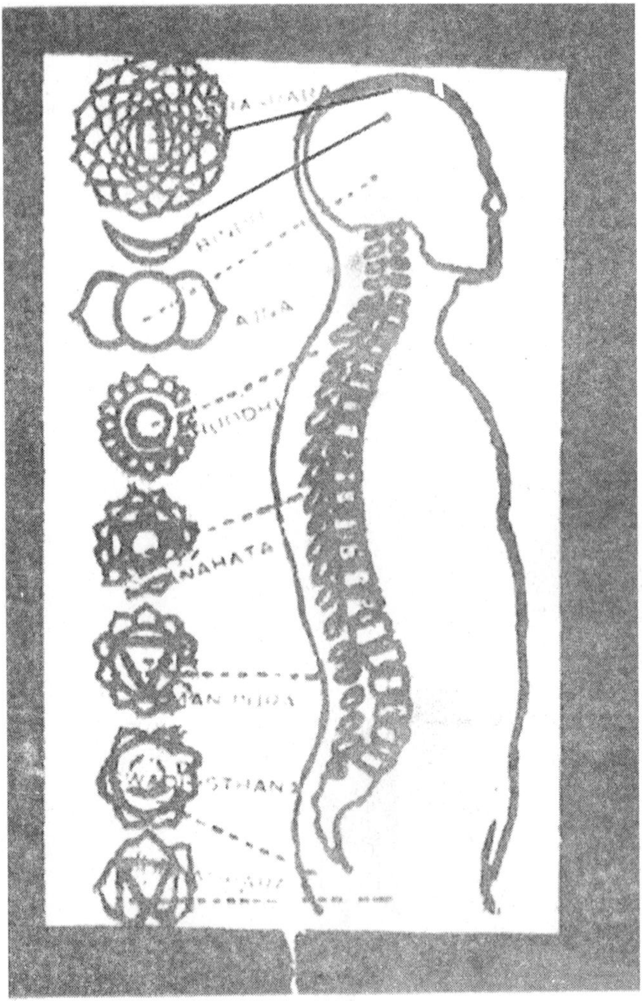

Eight Chakras (Upwards) अष्टचक्र

नीचे से ऊपर :
मूलाधार, स्वाधिष्ठान, मणिपुर, अनाहत, विशुद्धि, आज्ञा, मनश्चक्र (बिन्दु, चन्द्र, ललाट), सहस्रार, मेरुदण्ड में स्थित अदृश्य सुषुम्णा नाड़ी में ये चक्र हैं।

Muladhar, Svadhišthan, Mañipur, Anãhãta, Vishddhi, Ájnã, Manashchakra, Sahasrãra – these are suituated in the spinal cord.

Step I
Moral Discipline

41
Moral Conduct

Yoga is a spiritual way of life. The purpose of Yoga is self-realisation. The Upanishads declare "ÃTMÃNAM VIDHI, i.e., "Know Thyself". The Bible also calls upon man: "Know Thyself". This can only be achieved by spiritual elevation, moral conduct of which is the sine qua non. We are all the time busy in meeting our physical and material requirements but that is just to live like an animal. Man is different from animal because of its rational and moral behaviour. Compassion, service of humanity, non-violence, truthfulness, honest living, non-covetousness and dedication to God elevate man spiritually. One must curb the baser instincts like hatred, jealously, greed, lust, anger and pride, and adopt the rational, moral and spiritual attitude in life.

To achieve this, Swami Vivekananda has advised, "If there is a change of heart and a change of values, then our daily life itself becomes divine life. Normally, we live in a fool's paradise with our scale of values tilted in favour of sense pleasures." This change of attitude will bring a metamorphosis in our being. Rudyard Kipling has said "If your being is right, your doing cannot possibly go wrong."

To inculcate spiritual lifestyle, there is a prayer in Rig Veda (5.51.11): SVASTI PANTHÃMANU CHAREMA SURYACHANDRA MASÃVIVA (122), i.e., we may incessantly follow the path of well-being of others, as do the Sun and the Moon. Albert Einstein has expressed the same sentiment, "Only a life lived for others is worth living." Renowned spiritualist Deepak Chopra has said, "The whole cosmos is your teacher. All that you need to do is to learn to listen."

Service of humanity is the service of God. Spiritual attitude in life will provide you peace and tranquility in life and help in meditation.

42
Treat Others Like Thyself

For one's moral upliftment and for treading the righteous path as also to ensure that one does not harm anyone, one must adopt the golden dictum: TAT TAVAMASI, i.e., thou art that. This means all beings are alike; each one has a noble Soul in him as yours. In the Upanishads, there is a dictum: 'ÃTMAVAT SARVABHÛTEŠU'. That means: "Treat all beings as yourself." The Mahabharata also states: ÃTMANAH PRATIKÛLÃNI PAREŠÃM NA SAMÃCHARET (124), i.e., what is adverse to you, do not enact on others. It serves as a beacon under the light of which one can never do anything wrong. Similar command we find in the Bible, "Do unto others as you wish to be done unto you." Talmud has also advised, "What is hateful to you, do not do to your fellow man. That is the law: All else is commentary."

Would you like somebody cheating you? No. Do not cheat anybody else. Would you like somebody harming you mentally or physically? No. Do not harm anybody in any way. Would you like somebody helping you when you are in need? Certainly yes. Always extend a helping hand to those who are in need.

Following this golden rule of treating others as yourself is the sure way to tread the right path. It will give you peace and make you progress in spiritual life.

The Universally Acknowledged Golden Rule

What is repugnant to you, do not act against others.
—Mahabharta 3000 BC

Do not do unto others all that which is not well for ourselves.
—Zoroastrianism 1000 BC

What you don't want done to yourself, don't do to others.
—Confucius 6th Century BC

Hurt not others with that which pains thyself
—Buddha 5th Century BC

In happiness and suffering, in joy and grief, we should regard all creatures as we regard our own self.
—Mahavira 5th Century BC

Do unto others as thou wish to be done unto you.
—The Holy Bible

No one of you is a believer until he desires for his brother which he desires for himself.
—Quran Sharif

43
Follow the Dictates of Your Conscience

Another sure way to spiritual elevation is to follow the dictates of one's conscience. God has provided all with Divine Spark called Conscience which always guides us as to what is right and what is wrong. While doing a thing, if you have a sense of fear or sense of shame, it is certain that that action is wrong and must not be performed. It is common knowledge that when a thief commits a theft, he always looks around whether anybody is seeing him and is afraid of being caught. This sense of fear which emanates from his conscience is indicative of the fact that that action is wrong. Similarly, while doing any particular thing, you feel happy and encouraged and you want that more and more people should come to know about your action, that thing is right and must be performed. Commenting on this natural phenomenon, Swami Dayanand has said that the entity that feels fear and shame or happiness and enthusiasm is the Soul and the entity that evokes these feelings is God. There is a *Mantra* in the Yajur Veda (19.77) to this effect: ASHRADDHÃM ANRITE ADADHÃT SHRADDHÃM SATYE PRAJÃPATIH (35), i.e., God has placed (in Soul) faith in Truth and aversion to Untruth.

A Sufi Saint has also expressed the same sentiment:

> "A touchstone God hath placed in every heart
> It separates, with surety, False from True."

The following statements of renowned luminaries are worthy of attention for action:

(i) "When I do good, I feel good.
When I do bad, I feel bad.

That is my religion."

— Abraham Lincoln

(ii) "Know only that what is moral is what you feel good after and what is immoral is what you feel bad after."

— Ernest Hemmingway

(iii) "Ignite your minds to pay heed to conscience.
Conscience is the light of the Soul that burns
Within the chambers of our psychological heart.
It protests whenever anything unrighteous
is done or thought of."

— Dr. A.P.J. Abdul Kalam

(iv) "Conscience is the mother-in-law whose visits never end."

— H.L. Menchen

Voice of conscience is considered to be the voice of God. Always follow the dictates of your conscience and you will never err.

Thus Spake Scholars on Vedas

The Vedas are the most post modern thing I have read.

—Vendy Doniger (American Indologist)

"The great Vedas – the most remarkable works containing not only religious ideas for a perfect life, but also facts which all the science has since proved true. Electricity, Radium, Electrons, Air Ships all seem to be known to the seers who found the Vedas."

—Mrs. Wheeler Willox

44
Think about the Opposite or Adverse Consequences

To follow the spiritual path is the most difficult thing to do. The scriptures of all the religions call upon us to control our anger, lust, greed, jealously, hatred and the like. But it is the most difficult thing to control such emotions and instincts. That is why, the saying 'Easier said than done'. Although difficult, controlling such emotions is not impossible. After all, Sages and Seers have controlled such emotions. Sage Patanjali has suggested one effective method: VITRAK BÃDHANE PRATIPAKŠA BÃDHANAM (13), i.e., one must develop an attitude of countering evil thoughts by invoking opposite feelings. For example, when one is over-powered by the emotion of anger, one must think that fire cannot be put out by fire, it can be put out only by water. So, calmness must be generated to control anger. One may divert one's attention from the situation and have three deep breaths. It will calm down the anger. In the case of lustful feeling about a beautiful person, one may visualise an ugly face or that of one's mother or sister; ill thoughts will disappear. In the face of temptation of stealing, say, by evading payment of government taxes or accepting bribe or tempted to make adulterations in food or medicines, practitioner may think of being caught and put in jail. In similar other situations, the practitioner may think of how will he feel if his friends and relatives and those whom he loves come to know of his despicable behaviour. He may also think of the plight of his children and other family members who are dependent on him for support; how will they manage their finances and cope with the taunts of their neighbours.

Alternatively, he may ponder over the arduous journey he has undertaken in the progress of Yoga *Sadhana*. He may visualise himself as an ardent Yoga practitioner, for above the ordinary men. He may curse himself for allowing such nefarious thoughts to crop up in his mind. He may have three deep breaths and recite mentally the name of God.

By invoking such feelings of adverse consequences, the evil thoughts will vanish and the practitioner will be spared from indulging in any wrong-doings.

The Practice of the Presence of God

"I cannot imagine how religious persons can live satisfied without the practice of the presence of God. Let it be your business to keep the mind in the presence of the Lord. If it sometimes wanders and withdraws itself from Him, do not much disquiet yourself for that: trouble and disquiet serve rather to distract the mind than to recollect it; the will must bring it back in tranquillity."

—Brother Lawrence

45
Be Always Mindful of Death and God

Spiritual elevation can also be achieved by always keeping in mind the possibility of one's death at any time and the existence of God who is Omnipresent, Omniscient and Dispenser of Justice. We are always engaged in amassing wealth and adding to material resources for our comfort as if we were to live forever. Regarding death, Ivern Ball has said, "Most of us can read the writing on the wall. We just assume it's addressed to someone else." We even do not mind depriving others of their rights in the pursuit of our comforts. One must always think that life is short and at any time, one can meet death, and that all the material wealth would remain here unutilised by him. One must, therefore, always do those deeds which are just and pious. Evil deeds always bring evil results. While doing anything which is wrong, one must always realise that there is some power which is present and seeing his bad deeds and the bad deeds will always return to him in one form or the other. The following noble thoughts should always be kept in mind:

(i) DVAU SANNIŠADYA YANMANTRAYETE
RÃJÃ TAD VEDA VARUÑAS TRITÎYAH (125)

— Atharva Veda (4.16.2)

(When two persons make any conspiracy, the third, God, knows that.)

(ii) "Thou compassest my path and my lying down and art acquainted with all my ways. For there is not a word in my tongue, but lo O Lord, Thou knowest it altogether. Whither shall I go from Thy spirit? Or whither shall I flee from Thy presence?"

— The Holy Bible (Psalms 139.3,4,7)

(iii) "First then fear God: for His fear is wisdom
And being wise, thou canst not err."

— Miguel Cervantes

(iv) "He that fearth Him and worketh
Righteousness is accepted of Him."

— St. Peter

(v) "We are all serving a life sentence, good behaviour is our only hope for a pardon."

— Dong Horton

(vi) "To him that soweth righteousness shall be sure reward.
Men do not gather grapes of thorns or figs of thistles.
The wages of sin is death and God will render to everyone according to their deeds."

— The Holy Bible

(vii) "These deeds of yours shall, verily, be brought back unto you, as if you were yourself the author of your own just punishment."

— Hadis: Sayings of Prophet Muhammad

It is our good or bad deeds which follow us after death and determine our future life. We must always pray to God to ward us off bad deeds.

Thus Prayed St. Peter

May the strength of God pilot us!
May the wisdom of God instruct us!
May the hand of God protect us!
May the word of God direct us!

46
Inculcate Feelings of Detachment

The cardinal principle for spiritual development is: TATRA SUKHAM YATRA NIVRITTIH , i.e., there is happiness where there is detachment. Therefore, for spiritual elevation, one must develop a feeling of detachment. The cause of suffering is our attachment to the worldly things. We are attached to things which give us pleasure and feel miserable when we lose them. The pleasure which these things give us is momentary and is only sensory pleasure and not everlasting bliss. It is stated in the Hindu Scriptures that if all the pleasures of the world are given to one person, he will not be happy because the material things are not capable of providing happiness. We know from experience that Kings or Rulers who have all the wherewithal of enjoyment and sensory pleasures are not really happy. In the pursuit of these pleasures, one also commits wrongs which subsequently make him miserable.

Too much attachment with children and family members which blinds one's sense of evenness is also not desirable. To look after one's family and their needs, evasion of taxes, taking bribes, cheating, theft or depriving others of their rights are often considered justifiable by spiritually blind people. While looking after one's children and family members is a duty, blinding attachment (*Moha*) to family relationships and craving for ensuring more comfortable life for them, by fair or foul means, is immoral and should always be shunned.

Contentment in life is essential. Benjamin Franklin said, "Who is rich? He that is content." Discontentment leads to high blood pressure, hypertension and other diseases apart from distraction in spiritual progress. Detachment will bring contentment and peace of mind.

Ramakrishna Paramhansa advised his disciples, "Do not let your cat come between you and your God." 'Cat' is the symbol of earthly belongings and beings with whom one is too much attached. Ralph Waldo Emerson has also said, "If a man owns land, the land owns him." So, for spiritual progress, inculcating detachment is necessary.

Mahatma Buddha advised his disciples to ponder over the following five facts of life which will lead them to Vairagya (Detachment)

(i) Sooner or later, old age will beset me, I cannot avoid it.

(ii) Sooner or later, disease will overpower me, I cannot avoid it.

(iii) Sooner or later, death will overtake me, I cannot avoid it.

(iv) All things that are dear to me are perishable and will, sooner or later, desert me. I cannot avoid it.

(v) I am shadow of my deeds, good or bad; I am responsible for them, I cannot avoid it.

When one ponders over these facts of life, tendency to acquire more and more things is weakened and his excessive attachment (*Moha*) to dear ones is also lessened. One also refrains from doing bad deeds. This leads him develop a feeling of detachment (*Vairagya*) which helps him become poised, composed and in attaining steady progress in meditation.

Science and Spirituality

'Do you not see whither science is tending? The Hindu nation proceeded through the study of the mind, through metaphysics and logic. The European nations start from external nature, and now they, too, are coming to the same results. We find that, searching through the mind, we at last come to that Oneness, that universal One, the internal Soul of everything, the essence and reality of everything. ... Through material science, we come to the same Oneness.'

—Swami Vivekananda

47
Self-Introspection (*ÃTMA – NIRÎKŠAÑ*)

One of the most effective methods of spiritual elevation is Self-Introspection. The foregoing methods of Moral Conduct – treating others as oneself, listening to the voice of the conscience, etc. are extremely helpful in raising one's spiritual level. But constant watch has to be kept whether one is actually following these guidelines or not; whether or not one was able to ward off evil thoughts by pondering over the adverse consequences of the intended action. For this, self-introspection is very essential.

While going to bed at night, one must mentally go through one's activities of the day and ask oneself pertinent questions whether one violated the voice of the conscience or did anything which was ethically wrong. If the answer is yes, one must resolve not to do it again.

One must also pray: VISHVÃNI DEVA SAVITAR DURITÃNI PARÃ SUVA YAD BHADRAM TANNA Ã SUVA (126), i.e., O God, whatever are my weaknesses, remove; and whatever is good for me, provide.

It is likely that during the course of the day, somebody might have offended you, hurt you or done something wrong to you, do not harbour any ill-will against him and submit yourself to the judgement of God and pray: YO ASMÃN DVEŠTI YAM VAYAM DUŠMASTAM VO JAMBHE DADHMAH (127), i.e., O God! One who has ill-will towards us or we who have ill-will towards someone, submit him and us to Your Jaws of Justice.

Stricto sensu, Self-Introspection is looking inwards, searching one's heart. It is a spiritual exercise. Carl Jung has said, "He who looks outwards, dreams. He who looks inwards, awakes." Self-Introspection makes you aware of your weaknesses and provides you a tool to correct yourself and, thereby, progress spiritually.

There are only two entities who know what you do or think. One, yourself and the other, God. No other person can know your thought processes and, therefore, cannot advise you how to correct yourself. Swami Vivekananda has succinctly stated, "You have to grow from the inside out. None can teach you, none can make you spiritual. There is no other teacher but your own Soul."

To achieve this goal, Self-Introspection is the unique and unfailing tool.

Thus Spake Plotinus

If in this retirement into thyself, "thou dost not yet find beauty there, do like a sculptor who chisels ...... So thou chisel away from thy soul what is superfluous, straighten that which is crooked, purify and enlighten what is dark and do not cease working at thy statue until virtue shines before thine eyes with its divine splendour and thou seest temperance seated in thy bosom with its holy purity."

48

Complete Control over Senses (*Pratyãhãr*)

Senses have a natural tendency of attraction towards sense objects like beauty, sound, taste. *Pratyãhãr* is Abstraction, i.e., after rigorous training, the senses shed their natural attraction, and become obedient servants of the Mind. Normally mind follows the senses, but now the senses follow the mind. Just as bees follow the queen bee, similarly the senses follow the dictates of the mind. The senses, now become inward-looking rather than outward-looking.

Control of the senses is not suppression of the senses, but sublimation of the senses. This is inculcated by being alert as to whether one is eating to live or living to eat. This is not to shut off senses of hearing or seeing, but to ensure the same are used for higher purpose. In *Pratyahar*, the abstraction is voluntary and the mind has no object of attraction in the external world, its field of activity is internal. Dr S. Radhakrishnan states in Indian Philosophy: "To hear the melodies of spirit, we must shut off noise of the world. This is not to renounce the powers of sight, hearing and speech. It is to open the inner eye to the spiritual realities, capture the sounds that come from the world of spirit, sing in silence the hymn of praise to the Supreme Being."

This state of mind is a bridge that leads to meditation. A Yoga Practitioner must attempt to withdraw senses from the outer world and focus on the inner world of peace and tranquillity.

Step II

Asana (Physical Exercises)

49
Instructions Regarding *Asana* and Health

- The purpose of *Asana* is to have a healthy mind in healthy body. Consequently, *Asanas* are of two types: one, useful for physical fitness and two, useful for meditation.
- For meditation, only 4 to 5 *Asanas* are suitable, viz., *Sukha Asana*, *Padma Asana*, *Ardhapadma Asana* and *Vajra Asana*. Any one of these *Asanas* in which one can sit errect comfortably for a long duration of time, without movement, may be practised and perfected. When someone is unwell and is not in a position to sit comfortably for meditation, one can do meditation in a Dead-Body Posture (*Shav-Asana*).
- *Hatha* Yoga has devised numerous *Asanas* for physical fitness. These are often named after the physical form of birds and animals. There is no need to do all the *Asanas*. Only 8 to 10 *Asanas* carefully selected could serve the purpose. One *Asana* may be practised for 2 to 3 minutes. The total duration of the *Asanas* should be half-an-hour or so.
- The *Hatha* Yoga *Asanas* are not part of the Patanjali Yoga System, but have been included here as these are helpful in keeping the body fit. Surely, good health is necessary for practising Yoga.
- After all the *Asanas*, *Shava Asana* – Dead Body Posture – must be practised. This will relieve all the fatigue and exertion and one could feel quite fresh and relaxed.
- In illness or in extreme fatigue, *Asanas* should not be practised. Only the *Shava Asana* should suffice and will give relief.

- Persons suffering from heart disease, high blood pressure, slip disc, spondylitis and pregnant women should consult Yoga expert before practising any *Asana*.
- While practising *Asanas*, if there is yawning, sneezing, etc., it should not be suppressed.
- *Asanas* should not be practised immediately after taking food or liquid. There should be a gap of at least 4 hours after food and about one hour after taking milk, juice, etc.
- Meat, alcohol and smoking should be avoided. This does not mean that if somebody eats meat or drinks, *Asanas* are prohibited for him. If these things are avoided, benefit will be more.
- Eating habits should be simple, the food should not be too spicy. Ayurvedic dictum is: Be '*Mit Bhogi*, *Hit Bhogi* and *Rit Bhogi*'. One should not eat too much. Always eat a bit less than required (*Mit Bhogi*). Don't eat junk food; Always eat nutritious food (*Hit Bhogi*). Always eat seasonal fruits and vegetables (*Rit Bhogi*). Follow the dictum: 'Drink food and eat water'. That means food should be properly chewed and water should be drunk slowly and not gulped. Dr. Samuel Johnson has stated "When diet is wrong, medicine is of no use. When diet is right, medicine is of no need."
- Food affects both the body and the mind. It is said YATHÃ ANNA TATHÃ MANA'. That means mind is as the food is. Honestly earned food brings peace. Food earned by dishonest means brings suffering to the mind.
- One must drink about two litres of water everyday. Do not drink water after food as it dilutes the secretions produced by the body for digestion at the time of taking food. Ayurvedic dictum is: BHOJNÃTE VIŠAM VÃRIH (128), i.e., after food, water is poison. One should not drink water in standing position.
- In the morning, take some medicinal things like ginger, lemon, garlic, aloe vera, amala and a few leaves of tulsi, neem and mint. These are helpful for relieving constipation and in warding off many diseases. Ayurveda's dictum is: SARVEŠÃMEVA ROGÃÑÃM NIDHÃNAM KOŠTHA

BADDHATÃ (129), i.e., constipation is the repository of all diseases.

- While practising *Asanas*, do not ignore half-an-hour of morning walk daily. Some thinker has said, "I have two doctors – one my right leg and the other my left leg." Always walk alone. That will provide relaxation to the mind. When walking in company, people tend to discuss office, business or family matters. That should be avoided. And don't forget to leave your mobile at home.

Thus Spake John K. Bangs

What fools indeed we mortals are
To lavish care upon a car.
With ne'er a bit of time to see
About our own machinery.

50
Meditation-Related *Asanas*

Sitting still in a comfortable posture, without movement, is *Asana*. For the purposes of meditation, the *Asana* should be extremely comfortable so that one does not get disturbed for sufficiently long period of time. During meditation, one should never sit in any difficult *Asana*. St. Augustine has said, "The comfort of the posture has much to do with the continuous stream of our meditation."

For meditation, *Sukha Asana* (Easy or Cross-legged Posture); *Padma Asana* (Lotus Posture); *Ardh-Padma Asana* (Half Lotus Posture), Siddha Asana or *Vajra Asana* (Rock or Kneeling Posture) are considered to be very comfortable. Researches have revealed that *Sukh Asana*, *Padma Asana,* etc. which resemble the shape of a pyramid, provide tranquillity. It has also been found that in Green Houses with pyramid shape, plants grew plentifully than in Green Houses in other shapes.

Sukh Asana is sitting in cross-legged position in which the right leg is kept under the left thigh and left leg under the right thigh. The palms, facing upwards, are to be placed on the knees, the index finger should touch the first bend of the thumb. Alternatively, palms, one on the other, could be placed on the lap.

In *Padma Asana*, the right foot is put on the left thigh and left foot on the right thigh, whereas in the *Ardh Padma Asana*, one foot is on the thigh and the other foot is under the thigh. The position of the palms should be as indicated in *Sukh Asana*.

In *Siddha Asana*, heel of the left foot is to be kept between the anus and the sex-organ and the heel of the right foot is to be kept above the sex-organ. Pressure is not to be exerted on the sex-organ. Both the heels should be below and above the sex-organ. The palms should be either on the knees or in the lap as in *Sukh Asana*.

In *Vajra Asana*, one is to kneel down and sit on the parted heels. One can sit on the floor, with the legs bent backward. The palms should be resting on the knees in downward position. Those who cannot sit in any of the cross-legged postures, find this *Asana* quite comfortable.

In all the above *Asanas*, one should sit straight. The spine, the head, the neck and the trunk should be in a straight line. There should be no movement. Place of *Asana* should be solitary clean, airy, even, neither hard nor cushy.

While sitting in any of the above *Asanas*, one should close one's eyes and think of the limitless sky or omnipresent God. Mind should be stilled and relaxed. After taking a few deep breaths, one should do meditation. When one attains perfection in *Asana*, one will not feel any thirst or hunger; heat or cold for a long time.

Yogic Posture

There, setting hard his mind upon The One,
Restraining heart and senses, silent, calm,
Let him accomplish Yoga, and achieve
Pureness of soul, holding immovable
Body and neck and head, his gazed absorbed
Upon his nose-end rapt from all around,
Tranquil in spirit, free of fear, intent
Upon his Bramcharya vow, devout,
Musing on Me, lost in the thought of Me.
That Yogin, so devoted, so controlled,
Comes to the peace beyond – My peace, the peace
Of high Nirvana!

—Sir Edwin Arnold
(The Song Celestial)
(Shrimad Bhagvad Gita – 6.13-15)

51
Health-Related *Asanas*

'You are the Temple of God', says the Bible. Famous poet Kalidasa has said: 'SHARÎRAM ADYA KHALU DHARMA SÃDHANAM' (9), i.e., this body is the means of spiritual advancement. It is through the body alone that we can render service to humanity. If the body is not fit, we cannot render any help to others, rather become dependent on others. If the body is aching, we cannot sit for meditation. So, to keep our body fit is our bounden duty.

The *Hatha* Yoga has devised various *Asanas* to keep the body fit. These *Asanas* are purported to give exercise to various parts of the body – the spine, the stomach, the chest, the neck, legs and arms. By doing these *Asanas*, the digestive, respiratory, spinal and blood-related problems are removed. Insomnia, psychosomatic problems, hypertension and heart-related problems are also removed by practising these *Asanas*.

Out of the eighty-four *Asanas* of *Hatha* Yoga, 10 *Asanas* have been selected which cover all parts of the body. However, while *Shîrsh-Asana* (Head Posture) and *Surya Namskar* are extremely beneficial for health but owing to paucity of space, these have not been included as many photographs of different positions are required to be carried to demonstrate these *Asanas*. All the same, at the end of this section, their benefits have been highlighted to encourage the practitioners to learn these *Asanas* from a Yoga expert. Practice of these 8 to 10 *Asanas* everyday for half-an-hour, will keep the practitioners healthy.

While the procedures of practising the selected 10 *Asanas* are indicated in the following lessons, in this lesson, the method of doing *Shava Asana* only is given. This *Asana* must be done for 5 minutes after practising other *Asanas*.

Lie down on your back like a dead body. The body should be straight. The neck and the head straight, not bent either side. The heels should be about six inches apart and the hands should be about 3-4 inches away from the thighs. The palms should be open and facing upwards. Breathe normally. Don't allow extraneous thoughts to come to your mind. Think only about your body. Mentally visit all the parts of the body – the head, the eyes, the ears, the throat, the lungs, the heart, the navel region, the pelvic region, the arms, the palms, the legs, knees, the feet and the toes. Imagine that energy is flowing to each part of the body. Those who believe in God, may pray for the proper functioning of all these parts.

Total relaxation will descend on the body. The exertion of *Asanas* will disappear. You will feel absolutely fresh and energised. This *Asana* is particularly useful for hypertension, high blood pressure, heart disease, backache and extreme fatigue. The aged and the sick can also do meditation in this *Asana*.

Vedic Nectar

Ã YANMÃ VENÃ ÃRUHANN
RITASYAM EKAMÃSÎNAM
HARYA TASYA PRIŠTHEH

—Rig Veda 8.100.5

On Me, who is seated in the yogic posture,
light of truth has started descending

52
Dhanur Asana (Bow Posture)

Lie on your belly. Catch hold of your ankles with respective hands. Breathe in and raise your head and trunk as high as possible, making the shape of a bow, with spine curved backwards. Ensure your knees are raised and do not touch the ground. The weight of the body should be on the navel region. You can also rock in this position. Short inhalations and exhalations should be taken during the rocking. Inhale when you go up and exhale as you come down.

This *Asana* gives adequate massage to the abdominal muscles and adds flexibility to the spine. The chest and neck are also exercised. This *Asana* is helpful in removing indigestion, gastric trouble, acidity, respiratory problems, spinal problems. This *Asana* is also helpful for cervical spondylosis. This *Asana* should be repeated for a few moments after *Hal Asana* and *Pashchimottan Asana*. People suffering from hernia and pregnant women should not do this *Asana* or *Bhujanga Asana* or any other *Asana* requiring stretching of abdominal muscles.

53

Bhujanga Asana (Cobra Posture)

Lie on your abdomen. Keep both legs together with heels up, toes touching the ground. Place the palms downward close to the shoulders. Breathe in and slowly raise your head and trunk with the least amount of pressure on the arms. The weight of the body should lie on the navel and not on the arms as Cobra does not have arms. Repeat this exercise three to four times. When you go up, inhale and when you come down, exhale and hold the breath while maintaining the pose. The beginners need not hold the breath. This exercise is adequate for 2-3 minutes.

In the *Asana*, the chest and neck muscles are properly flexed. This exercise is good for respiratory problems, backache and problems related with thyroid gland. It is also beneficial for persons suffering from cervical spondylosis. People suffering from hernia or pregnant women should not do this *Asana*.

54

Pashchimottan Asana (Forward- Bending Posture)

Sit with both legs stretched forward. Gradually exhale. Raise your hands. Keeping your hands stretched, bend your head and trunk over the legs. Try to catch the toes of your feet. The elbows should be bent and touching the ground and head should touch the knees. The legs should remain completely stretched without raising the knees. The body should be bent forward as low as possible. It is a difficult *Asana.* If the head does not touch the knees, don't bother. Keep the head as close to the knees as possible. Hold the position as comfortable and repeat two to three times. Doing this *Asana* for 2-3 minutes is adequate. After this *Asana*, do *Dhanur Asana* for a few moments.

This *Asana* exercises the abdominal muscles, the spine, shoulders, arms, legs, eyes and neck. This *Asana* is useful for all the organs in the stomach, spine-related problems, arthritis, insomnia. Persons suffering from cervical spondylosis, hernia and pregnant women should not do this *Asana*.

55

Matsya Asana (Fish Posture)

Sit in *Padma Asana* (Lotus Posture) or *Sukha Asana* (Cross-legged Posture). Lean backwards. Rest your hands and then forearms on the ground. Bring your arms back and firmly placing your hands on the ground, raise your chest as high as possible, bending the head backwards. The weight of the body should rest on the hips and the middle part of the head. Lift your hands off the ground and catch the toes of the feet with respective hands. Breathe normally. Hold the position as long as comfortable. While releasing the posture, hold the breath. First release the toes and bring the arms back on the ground. With their support, bring the head and the back on the ground, Now exhale and rise with the help of elbows and release the lotus or crossed-leged posture. Alternatively, release the posture in the lying down position. This *Asana* provides flexibility to the spine by backward bending. It is useful for digestive and respiratiory systems, thyroid- and spine-related problems. Mentally visualise that all the related parts of the body are being energised. After the *Matsya Asana*, perform *Pashchimottan Asana* for one minute. Hernia patients and pregnant women should not do this *Asana*.

56
Ardhamatsyendra Asana (Spinal Twist Posture)

Stretch the legs in front of you. Bend the right leg and place the right heel close to the anus. Raise the left knee, keeping the foot flat on the ground at the right side of the left knee. Now stretch the right hand forward across the raised left knee and try to catch the thumb of left foot. Stretch the left arm at the back in horizontal position. Swing the trunk and neck to the left and look towards the left. Breathe normally. Hold this position for 2 minutes or as comfortable. Unlock the posture and repeat it by interchanging the position of the arms, legs and neck.

This *Asana* exercises the whole body, the spine, the back, the legs, the arms, the neck, the eyes and the abdomen. It gives flexibility to the spine and removes backaches, gastric trouble, constipation, problems of arthritis, cervical spondylosis. Mentally visualise that all these organs are being energised. Pregnant women should not do this Asana.

57

Gomukh Asana (Cow-Head Posture)

Sit in cross-legged position. Bring the left heel under the anus and sit on the heel. Place the right leg over the left leg keeping the heel as close to the left hip as possible. Raise the left arm and bend it from the elbow and put the hand at the back. Put the right arm also at the back. Interlock the fingers of both the hands. The left elbow should be in the vertical position and the left arm should be touching the ear. The back should be erect and neck straight. Breathe normally. Hold the posture for 2 minutes or as comfortable. Unlock the posture and repeat it by interchanging the position of the legs and arms. This *Asana* exercises the shoulders, the neck, the arms and the back. Backaches and cervical problems are removed.

58
Makar Asana (Crocodile Posture)

Lie on the belly. Breathe in and raise your head. Keep the elbows on the ground and rest your face in the cups of the palms. Raise your legs with knees touching the ground. The knees should be 3-4 inches apart and the feet should touch each other. Normal breathing may be done during the posture. A bit of exercise of the knees can also be done in this *Asana*. Stretch the right leg, the toes should touch the ground. Bend the left leg, heel should touch the buttock. Legs should go up and down alternately. Do this 10-12 times.

This *Asana* provides exercise to the stomach, chest, arms, legs and knees. It helps in removing gastric problem, obesity and other problems related with stomach. It provides increased blood supply to the knees, removes pain of the knee joints and elbow joints. It is a very restful *Asana* and can be done up to 10 minutes. To relieve fatigue of the day or of that of the difficult *asanas*, this *asana* can be done.

The *Asana* is useful for ladies after delivery. Children of 2-3 years of age can be made to lie in this *Asana* for 2-3 minutes, 2-3 times a day. It will remove their stomach problems, gastric and urinary problems. It may be ensured that they do not lie in this posture after taking milk.

59

Sarvãnga Asana (All-Limbs Posture)

This is a posture in which nearly all parts of the body are exercised. That is why it is called *Sarvãnga Asana.* Lie flat on your back with hands alongside your body. With the palms resting on the ground, gently lift the legs upwards. Now let the hands support the back at the hips, with the elbows resting on the ground. Then push your body further up, raising the legs straight making a right angle. Support the body by the hands from the middle of the back. The weight of the body should rest on the shoulders and the arms. The head should rest on the ground and the chin should touch the chest.

The *Asana* may be done for 3 minutes or as comfortable. Breathing should be normal during the posture. To unlock the posture, gently bend legs towards the head, release the support of the hands from the back and slowly bring down the trunk and the legs and lie on the back. Then rise.

This *Asana* exercises the shoulders and the thyroid gland, makes the spine elastic. The blood circulation is more in the neck region and the head. This *Asana* improves eye-sight, removes dyspepsia, constipation, gastro-intestinal disorders. It also cures leprosy. This *Asana* has nearly all the benefits of *Shirsha Asana* (Head Posture).

60
Hala Asana (Plough Posture)

Lie on the back as in *Sarvãnga Asana*. Lift the body upwards with palms resting on the ground. Keep the legs together and push these further over your head. Keep the arms firmly on the ground and keep on bending the legs forward until the toes touch the ground. Exhalation will help in bending the legs over the head. The legs should be straight, toes touching the ground. The arms should also be straight in parallel position in the opposite direction and palms touching the ground. The chin should touch the chest. The weight of the body should rest on the shoulders and the neck. Breathing should be normal during the posture. This posture should be retained for 2-3 minutes or as comfortable.

Unlock the posture by gently raising the legs up and then backwards down. Support of the hands to the back may be taken, if necessary.

This posture flexes the spine, the shoulders, the arms, the neck, the chest and muscles of the stomach. This exercise is useful for digestive, respiratory, spinal and thyroid-related problems. While doing the *Asana*, visualise that the said parts of the body are being energised. After this *Asana*, do *Dhanur Asana* for a few moments.

Heart disease patients should consult a Yoga expert before doing this *Asana*. Persons suffering from high blood pressure, cervical spondylosis, slip disk or hernia, TB of the spine, liver problem and pregnant women should not practise this *Asana*.

61

Shîrša-Asana (Head Posture)

Shiršha Asana is the king of all *Asanas*. In this *Asana*, the whole body rests on head. That is why, it is called Head Posture, upside down posture. In this *Asana*, the blood supply to the head is maximum. All the nerves of the brain and the head region get toned up. This sharpens the memory, improves eyesight and wards off diseases related to the nervous system.

Medical science also recognises the benefits of the Head Posture. In medical terminology, it is known as Inversion Therapy. Over 2,400 years ago, Hippocrates propagated Inversion Therapy. Under this treatment, a patient was hung upside down, tied to a ladder. In the modern times, Dr. Robert Marten prescribed this therapy to the American soldiers in 1960. In the Inversion Therapy, the legs were tied and the soldier was hung upside down. The medical doctors opine that this posture supplies ample amount of blood to the brain and the flow of energy is also reversed for a few moments, which is very beneficial for health.

We could not include *Shiršah Asana* in our book owing to paucity of space. Explaining the *Shiršah Asana* involves many postures along with their photographs. So, it has been left out, but this does not mean a practitioner should not practise it. This *Asana* is extremely beneficial and is highly recommended, but should be learnt from an expert in Yoga, otherwise one may get hurt. A person suffering from high blood pressure and epilepsy should not do this *Asana*. Those who cannot do this *Asana*, must do *Sarvang Asana*.

62

Surya (Isha) Namaskar Asana (Salutation to God)

Out of the 84 *Asanas* propounded by the *Hatha* Yoga, three are very prominent and effective. These are: *Shiršaha Asana*, *Sarvang Asana* and *Surya Namaskar Asana*. We have already dealt with the first two.

Surya Namaskar Asana like the other two energises the whole body. It involves many postures. Owing to space constraints, it is not possible here to demonstrate how to perform this *Asana*. As it energises the whole body, it wards off many diseases related to the spine, stomach, thyroid gland, arthritis, et al. It is, therefore, recommended that this *Asana* must be learnt and performed by all the practitioners of Yoga.

It is unfortunate that the Yoga Capsule devised by the Ayusha Ministry for the International Day of Yoga Celebrations, *Surya Namaskar Asana* has been excluded, whereas, in many countries, it forms a prominent part of the Yoga demonstration on this day celebrated by almost all the countries in the world including the Muslim countries.

Some of the adherents of Islam in our country refrain from doing *Surya Namaskar Asana* as it amounts to obeisance to an object of Nature. Islam proclaims that only God is to be paid obeisance to (*Sajda*). The Rig Veda also proclaims: EK EVA NAMASYAH (42), i.e., only one is bowed to or worshipped.

We would like to clarify here that the word *Surya* in the *Surya Namsakar* does not mean Sun, but God. In the Vedas Indra, Varun, Surya, et al are all the names of God. Prof. Max Muller's following words in 'India: What Can It Teach Us' are worthy of attention: "They were all meant to express the Beyond, the Invisible behind the Visible, the Infinite within the Finite, the Supernatural above the Natural, the Divine, Omnipresent, Omnipotent."

Prof. Max Muller's above assertion is based on the internal evidence from the Vedas. The Yajur Veda (7.42) declares: SURYA ĀTMĀ JAGATAS-TAS THUŠASHCHA (131), i.e., SURYA is the Soul of all the animate and inanimate world. JAGAT literally means the moving Universe. How can our tiny Sun, which itself is Soul-less, can be the Soul of the vast universe comprising billions and billions of galaxies having trillions and trillions of suns? Obviously, here the word Sun means God.

It is not only the Vedas, but many religions and scholars declare God as the Soul of the Universe:

(i) The Universe is one stupendous Whole
Whose Body Nature is, and God the Soul.

— Alexandra Pope

(ii) HAK JANE JAHĀN ASTA
VA JAHĀN JUMLĀ BADAN

— Sufi Poet

i.e., God is the Soul of the Universe and
the whole Universe is His Body.

(iii) ALLĀH BE KULLE SHAMEEN MUHIT
ALLĀHO NÛR US SAMAVATI VAL ARD

— The Holy Quran

i.e., God encompasseth the whole world and pervades it.
His light enlightens the heavenly bodies and the earth.

(iv) God said let there be light
And there was light.

— The Holy Bible

In short, in *Surya Namaskar*, the word *Surya* means God. And He is worthy of being bowed to by all. The Holy Quran states: "O God! the Sun, the Moon, the Stars are working for us under your Command. Seeing these signs of Nature, we can surmise your might, wisdom and craftsmanship."

To avoid the controversy over *Surya Namaskar Asana*, our humble suggestion is that it be renamed as *Isha Namaskar Asana* as *Surya* here means God. It will obviate objection of our Muslim brethren as it means an *Asana* of *Sajda* to God, Salutation to God. If any prayer is necessary, let that be: SVASTI PANTHÃM-ANUCHAREM SURYÃ CHANDRA MASAVIVA (122), i.e., "O God! Give me strength to follow the path of service of humanity as do the Sun and the Moon incessantly.

Thus Spake a Sufi Poet

AÎ BAR-TAR AZ KHAYÃL
O QAYÃS O GUMÃN O WAHM
W-AZ HAR CHE GUFTA-EM
O SHANÎD-EM O KHWÃNDA-EM

(Thou art beyond all thought, conception, guess
Imagination, yea, and far beyond
All we have spoken, heard or read in books;
These deal with Objects –
Thou Subject of all!)

63

Šatkarma (Six Procedures)

Jal Neti (*Nasal Wash*), *Dhauti* (Chest Wash)

Hatha Yoga has propounded *Shatkarma* or *Shatkriya* for keeping the body clean and healthy. As the English word Action for *Karma* and Activity for *Kriya* do not convey the intended meaning here, we have used the medical term procedure, which conveys its real intent. *Shatkarma* – the six procedures are: *Neti*, *Dhauti*, *Vasti*, *Nauli*, *Tratak* and *Kapãl Bhãti*.

Tratak is an exercise for fixing attention and has been explained in lesson IV/2. *Kapãl Bhãti* is a breathing exercise and has been explained in lesson III/10. *Vasti* is a stomach wash and *Nauli* relates to churning of the intestines. Both are difficult exercises and should be learnt from some Yoga expert. The procedures for *Neti* and *Dhauti* are explained below.

Neti is of two types – *Jal Neti*, i.e., Nasal Wash by water and *Sutra Neti*, i.e., Nasal cleansing by thread. *Sutra Neti* is slightly difficult and should be learnt from a Yoga expert. *Jal Neti* is easy and could be done daily or atleast twice a week. This is as follows: A pot with a nozzle is available in the market for *Jal Neti*. Put some warm water with a bit of salt in it, hold it in your left hand. Tilt your neck rightwards, hold breath and pour water from the pot-nozzle into the left nostril, water will come out from the right nostril. Cleans the nostril. Tilt your neck leftwards; hold breath and hold the pot in the right hand and pour water from the pot-nozzle into the right nostril and water will come out from left nostril. Cleanse the nostril. Repeat this process 5-6 times. But ensure that you hold your breath while pouring water into either of the nostrils; otherwise water will land up in the mouth. In between, you can breathe normally. After the exercise, do *Kapãl Bhãti* and throw away the remnants of water from the nostril, otherwise the remaining water may cause headache.

Jal Neti cleans the nostrils. Dust particles and mucus, etc. are removed. Relieves the practitioner from sneezing, cold, etc. and helps him in doing the *Pranayama* properly.

Dhauti means act of washing. It is of two types – *Jal Dhauti*, water-washing and *Sutra Dhauti*, cloth-washing. *Sutra Dhauti* is difficult and should be learnt from a Yoga expert. *Jal Dhauti* is quite easy and should be done as follows:

After going to the toilet, drink about 8-10 glasses of warm water with a bit of salt. Walk a few steps. Stand straight and bend forward. Press the belly. Put two fingers in the mouth and press the root of the tongue and vomit. Drink 3-4 glasses of salted warm water again and repeat the process. This procedure will clean the food pipe, the chest and the stomach. Problems of cough, acidity, constipation, asthma and the like will be removed. Doing this exercise once in fortnight is adequate.

What is the real intent of *Shatkarma*?

Sage Patanjali has prescribed *Shaucha* (Purity/Cleanliness) in his five *Niyamas*. The obvious purpose of *Shatkarma* is cleansing the body, keeping it fit as also improving longevity. It has been said: KÃLAM VANCHANÃRTHÃYA KARMA KURVANTI YOGINÃH (132), i.e., for cheating Death, the Yogis perform *Shatkarma*. Swami Dayanand Saraswati was given poison 17 times; with the help of *Vasti* and *Nauli,* he washed the stomach and expelled the poison.

But the real intent of *Shatkarma* is the same what Sage Patanjali calls the fruit of *Shaucha*: SHAUCHÃT SVÃNGA-JUGUPSÃ PARAIR-ASANSARGAH (133) (Yoga *Darshana* II/40), i.e., from the physical purity arises disgust for one's own body and disinclination to come in physical contact with others. This falls within Yoga's overall purpose of *Purušа-Prakriti-Viyoga* – severance of relations between Soul and Body.

Step III

Prãñãyãma (Breathing Exercises)

64
Instructions Regarding *Pranayama*:

- Please go through the write-up on *Pranayama* under the section 'Constituents of Yoga'.
- *Pranayama* is an important part of the Yoga discipline. It may be noted that normal breathing is not *Pranayama*. Pranayama is regulated breathing. *Pranayama* means expansion of *Prana* (Energy) which these exercises provide. *Pranayama* exercises should be performed as per the instructions. Not following the instructions properly may cause some harm. Instructions given in this book are only indicative in nature. It will be more useful if some help of a Yoga expert is taken.
- *Pranayama* exercises should be performed by breathing through the nose and not by the mouth. There are some exercises which require breathing through the mouth. These have been separately indicated. All normal breathing at all times must be done through the nostrils. Nature has provided a bush or small hair in the nostrils which serve as a filter. All dust and other unwanted particles are thrown out through the process of sneezing which is automatically activated. Furthermore, in winter, cold air also gets warmed up before it reaches the lungs. Breathing through the mouth is harmful as dust and harmful particles as also cold air reach the lungs unobstructed. This is one of the major causes of tuberculosis.
- Even while sleeping, breathing should be through the nose and the face should never be covered with blanket as it obstructs the flow of fresh air. Breathing through the mouth at night will parch the throat and will cause snoring.

- *Pranayama* exercises should be done in the open in fresh air, facing the direction from which gentle breeze is blowing. If done in a room, the windows should be kept open. *Pranayama* exercises should not be performed in gale or facing the direction from which gust of wind is coming because it is likely to bring along the dust particles.
- Breathing exercises should be done around sunrise and sunset. If this time is not suitable, it may be done at any other time.
- One must cultivate the habit of deep breathing. Shallow breathing is the cause of many diseases, particularly tuberculosis. Dr. Fisher has stated in his book 'How to Live': "Take deep breathing exercises daily several times a day. A hundred deep breaths a day is a recipe for avoiding Tuberculosis."
- While walking, develop the habit of Ten-Step-Breathing, i.e., breathe-in for four steps, breathe-out for six steps. Don't hold the breath. Deep-breathing is not *Pranayama* and may be practised anytime for promoting health. It is beneficial because of increased intake of oxygen and of somewhat greater influx of *Prana* into the body. As it does not affect the *Pranic* Current in the body, its practice is not attended by any risk. Except this deep breathing, no *Pranayama* exercise is to be done while walking or doing anything. This may be harmful. All breathing exercises should be done while sitting steadily and comfortably. In Sage Patanjali's words: TASMIN SATI (Having attained that), i.e., perfection in *Asana*, *Pranayama* should be practised.
- Instructions regarding food given in Step II: *Asanas* should be followed for *Pranayama* also.
- Meat-eating, drinking and smoking should be avoided. Smoking is particularly harmful for respiratory system. All the same, *Pranayama* is not prohibited to those who drink, smoke or eat meat.
- Breathing exercises should be done empty stomach. These should not be done immediately after taking food or any liquid. There should be a gap of at least four hours after taking food and about an hour of taking liquid.

- Breathing exercises should not be done when one is ill. Only deep breathing would suffice.
- Breathing exercises should be done after the physical exercises/*Asanas*, the last of which should be *Shava Asana* (Dead Body Posture).
- If, while doing any breathing exercise, there is parch in the mouth or heaviness in the head or feeling of exertion in the body, the exercise should be stopped.
- *Pranayama* exercises are of two types: (i) for improving health; and (ii) helpful in meditation.
- The *Pranayama* exercises related to health may be done for 20-25 minutes and should be followed by *Shava Asana* (Dead Body Posture) for five minutes.
- The breathing exercises related to meditation may be done before sitting for meditation. About 10 minutes of meditation-related breathing exercises is adequate.
- *Pranayama* should be done with eyes closed and with each inhalation and exhalation, you could mentally recite 'AUM' and visualise that all diseases, weaknesses and bad thoughts are vanishing and good health, good thoughts, peace and tranquillity are enveloping you. One may also pray: AGNE YANME TANVÃ ÛNAM TANMA ÃPRIÑA (134), i.e. whatever shortcoming is in my body, remove it.

65
Meditation-Related *Trividha Pranayama*

Taitreya Ãranyaka says: TRIVRIT VAI PRÃNÃH (19), i.e., *Prana* has three tendencies. Yoga *Darshana* names these as *Bãhya Vritti* (Exhalation), *Abhyãntar Vritti* (Inhalation) and *Stambha Vritti* (Retention), holding the breath where it is. This is also called *Kumbhaka Vritti*. Inhalation is also known as *Pûraka* and Exhalation is also known as *Rechaka*.

Yoga *Darshana* also mentions fourth *Vritti* as *Bãhya-Ãbhyantar-Vishya-Akšhepi Chathûrthah (135)*, i.e., interrupting the two-way flow of *Prana* (Inhalation and Exhalation) is the Fourth *Pranayama*. The first three are known as *Trividh Pranyama*.

One may say that one first breathes in and then breathes out. Then why does Sage Patanjali first mention Exhalation and then Inhalation? This is so because while normally breathing out, one does not breathe out fully, some foul breath is left inside. In *Pranayama*, one has to first exhale completely, and throw out foul breath and then inhale.

This must be clarified here that only these four are Meditation-related *Pranayama* as per Sage Patanjali; All others are *Hatha Yoga Pranayama* aimed at improving health.

Trividh Pranayama makes breath prolonged and subtle.

Sit in *Sukha Asana*, *Ardh-Padma Asana*, *Padma Asana* or *Vajra Asana* as comfortable. Keep your eyes closed; recite the name of God, thinking of His attributes and visualise that peace and tranquillity are enveloping you. Now, do as follows:

A. *Abhyantar Kumbhak* (Internal Retention): First breathe out completely. Breathe in as deeply as possible up to the navel region.

The flow of the breath inside should be as smooth as one takes some juice with a straw without any obstruction. Retain the breath as long as you can comfortably. The moment you start feeling uncomfortable, breathe out. Forcible retention of breath is harmful. Now breathe out completely. This process is called *Abhyantar Kumbhak.*

Normal ratio in inhalation and exhalation is 1:2, i.e., if you take two seconds to breathe in, you should take four seconds to breathe out and retention should be four times of inhalation, that means eight seconds. So, the ratio of Inhalation (*Purak*), Retention (*Kumbhak*) and Exhalataion (*Rechak*) is 1:4:2. But this ratio should be attained gradually and should not be forced. If you feel uncomfortable in between, breathe normally.

It must be kept in mind that Kumbhak, i.e., Retention/Holding of Breath is an essential element of *Pranayama*, but it is also the source of danger in the practice of *Pranayama. Kumbhak* should be performed gently, not forcefully, and gradually, especially in internal *Kumbhak.*

B. *Bãhya Kumbhak* (External Retention): Exhale fully. Slightly contracting the anus and your stomach below the navel, throw out the breath completely as one vomits out and hold the breath as long as you can comfortably, and then inhale slowly. This completes the process of *Bahya Kumbhak.*

First the *Abhyantar* and the *Bahya Kumbhak* are to be done separately. After some practice, the two could be combined.

C. *Stambha Vritti* (Retention): This is the retention of breath wherever it is. Just be watchful of the breathing process. Hold the breath during inhalation or exhalation when neither is yet complete.

66
Meditation-Related *Chathurtha* (Fourth) *Pranayama*

Akshepak means Interference with Inhalation and Exhalation. This is also known as the Fourth *Pranayama*. This is a breathing process which is interrupted during inhalation and exhalation. First exhale completely. Now inhale upto the navel region and hold the breath. During retention you may mentally recite the Gayatri Mantra. Inhale further upto the chest, hold again. Inhale upwards upto the throat and hold again. When inhalation is complete, start exhaling. Exhale upto the chest and hold; exhale up to the navel and hold. And exhale further emptying the stomach completely and hold. Secondly, in the midst of inhalation or exhalation, reverse the process. This *Pranayama* is difficult and must be done with the help of some Yoga expert.

The Fourth *Pranayama* is also known as *Keval Kumbhak* or Natural Internal Retention of the Breath. This is that stage when in Meditation, the practitioner becomes forgetful of his breath and the breath is so minute and slow that it becomes difficult to know whether the practitioner is breathing or not.

It would be noted that retention is in all the four *Pranayamas*. In the first, inhalation is done completely as one drinks water with a straw and thereafter retention is done. In the second, exhalation is done completely as one vomits and empties the stomach and retention is done thereafter. In the third, *Stambha Vritti*, while inhaling or exhaling, retention is done suddenly. In the Fourth *Pranayama*, retention is done repeatedly during inhalation and exhalation. That is why, it is also called 'Ubhayãkšepi', i.e., two-way interrupting *Pranayama*.

Only four types of *Pranayama* are helpful in Meditation. The beginners should start only with the first three mentioned above: Inhalation (*Purak*); Exhalation (*Rechak*); and Retenion (*Kumbhak*) known as *Trividh Pranayama*. After a round of 3 to 7 times of this exercise, meditation should be started.

During breathing with composed mind, one would notice that while breathing in, sound of 'SO' is being emitted; And while breathing out, sound of 'HAM' is being emitted. That is, one complete breath emits the sound of 'SOHAM'. SOHAM means 'I am that'. I am that entity which is breathing. I am the entity different from the body that sustains the body. And if you drop S and H from the sound, you get the sound of OM. That means OM is sustaining me, spiritually inclined practitioners should meditate on OM.

Patanjali Yoga System speaks of only meditation-related *Pranayama* which has been explained above. Hereafter, all the *Pranayama* exercises are health-related exercises.

Thus Spake Mahatma Gandhi

A clean confession combined with a promise
not to commit the sin again,
when offered before one who has the right to receive it,
is the purest type of repentance.

67

Health-Related *Svar Parivartan* (Altering Breath) *Nadi Shodan* (Cleansing of Nerves) /*Anulom Vilom Pranayama*

Hatha Yoga has devised an elaborate system of *Asana* and *Pranayama* to imbue physical strength and energise the body to prevent and cure diseases. About *Asanas*, we have already explained. Out of the numerous *Pranyamas*, we have selected *Nadi Shodhan*, *Sûrya/Chandra* Bhedi, *Bhastrika*, *Kapãl Bhãti*, *Sheetali/Sheetkari*, *Ujayee*, *Bhramari*, *Traya Sthani* (Three-Stage Breathing) *Pranayama* and *Tartamyamaya Prãñayama* (Synchronised Breathing), which are explained below. All these are health-related *Pranyamas*.

Normally, we breathe either from the left nostril or from the right nostril. And this keeps on changing every hour or so. However, breathing through both the nostrils is an ideal condition which is reflective of perfect health.

This exercise is related to altering the breath, thereby cleansing the nervous system and the respiratory system and enabling one to breathe through both nostrils.

Right nostril breathing generates heat in the body and that is why it is called *Suryasvar* (Sun-breathing) and left nostril breathing causes cooling in the body and is known as *Chandraswar* (Moon-breathing). When one breathes through both the nostrils, it is called *Sushmnasvar* (spinal breathing). *Surya Svar* flows through *Ida Nadi* which is also known as *Ganga Nadi*. *Chandra Svar* flows through *Pingla Nadi* which is also known as *Yamuna Nadi*. And *Sushma Svar* flows through *Sushma Nadi* which is also known as *Saraswati Nadi*. Actions requiring energy like eating, playing, fighting should be performed during right nostril breathing and actions requiring calmness should be performed during left nostril breathing, e.g. singing, negotiations. The meditation worship or any other spiritual action should be done while breathing through both the nostrils.

Nadi Shodhan/Anulom-Vilom

Sit in a comfortable posture. Close your right nostril with your thumb. Inhale and exhale through the left nostril 3-4 times. Close your left nostril with your index finger and inhale as deeply as possible and exhale completely emptying the stomach through the right nostril 3-4 times. Now without closing any nostril, inhale, through the left nostril and exhale through the right nostril. Then inhale through the right nostril and exhale through the left nostril. Repeat this process 8-10 times. Normally, you should be able to inhale and exhale through alternate nostrils without closing either. If you find some difficulty initially, you may take the help of your thumb and index finger as advised above. Never close both the nostrils. Nor there is any need to retain the breath inside or outside. Now both the nostrils are properly cleansed and you can inhale and exhale through both the nostrils. This exercise is called *Nadi Shodan Pranayama*, i.e., Nerves Cleansing *Pranayama*. This is also known as *Anulom/Vilom Pranayama*. This exercise may be done for 5 minutes in summer and 10 minutes in winter. The other method of altering the breathing process is to lie on the left side to have right nostril breathing and on the right side left nostril breathing.

This exercise is extremely effective for cleansing nerves, blood, asthma, gastric problems, low and high blood pressure and in fever. It is also helpful for Rheumatism, Parkinsons' Disease, Neuro problems and Depression.

NB: This exercise should be done first and the other breathing exercises later.

68

Health-Related *Svar Parivartan Pranayama* (Altering Breath): *Sûrya Bhedi/Chandra Bhedi Pranayama*

Altering breath is an effective means of preventing/curing many diseases. When a person is having an attack of asthma disease, or having acute pain, he should observe which nostril is functioning at that time. Having spotted that, one must close that nostril and start breathing from the other nostril. After 15-20 minutes, he would feel some relief.

Persons suffering from low blood pressure should cultivate the habit of breathing through the right nostril. Persons suffering from high blood pressure should cultivate the habit of breathing through the left nostril. During high fever, breathe through the left nostril. During pneumonia, breathe through the right nostril. Breathing through both the nostrils is the perfect state of health. After practising this for a month or so, one may be cured of the disease.

For *Surya Bhedi* and *Chandra Bhedi Pranayama,* sit in a comfortable position. For *Surya Bhedi Pranayama*, inhale through the right nostril and exhale through the left nostril. *Surya Bhedi* generates heat in the body. In this *Pranayama*, *Kumbhak* (Retention) is also done.

Similarly, while practising *Chandra Bhedi Pranayama*, inhale through the left nostril and exhale through the right nostril. This *Pranayama* generates coolness in the body. In this *Pranyama*, Kaumbhak (Retention) is also done.

In one day, both the *Surya Bhedi* and the *Chandra Bhedi Pranayamas* are not advised.

69

Trideshi Pranayama (Three-Stage Breathing)

The so-called civilised people living in urban areas do not follow the natural way of breathing. Their breathing is normally quick and shallow. They breathe up to the throat and the lungs do not get fully exercised, which is responsible for many diseases. The *Trideshi Pranayama* (three-stage breathing) is breathing up to the navel region, chest region and throat region.

Sit in a comfortable posture. Close your eyes. Have three deep breaths and recite the name of God. Keep your thumbs on hip bones and your palms in horizontal position on your navel region, Breathe in deeply upto the navel region. Retain the breath for two to three seconds and breathe out. While you breathe in, your stomach should expand and while you breathe out, the stomach should contract. Repeat this process of inhalation and exhalation 6 to 8 times. Those who believe in God could mentally recite the name of God during inhalation and exhalation and during the retention period of two to three seconds, may mentally recite 'God is great and merciful' or AUM NAMOSHIVÃYA (I bow to God for my well-being).

Have 2 to 3 normal deep breaths. Now keep your thumbs under the armpits and the palms in the horizontal position on the chest. Breathe in up to the chest region, reciting mentally the name of God. Hold for a few seconds, reciting AUM NAMO SHIVAAY and exhale reciting AUM. Repeat this process 6 to 8 times.

Have 2 to 3 normal deep breaths. Now keep your palms on the back of your shoulders. The elbows should be above and the arms should be close to the ears. Inhale and exhale with the mental recitation of the name of God. Now inhalation and exhalation being short are exercising the upper part of the lungs. In between, hold the breath for a few seconds and recite AUM NAMO SHIVÃYA. Repeat this process 6 to 8 times. Breathe normally 2 to 3 times.

During all the three stages of the exercise, mentally visualise that all the toxins, diseases, infirmities of the body are being flushed out and the strength, vitality and peace are descending in the body. This exercise is now complete.

This exercise provides complete breathing and nourishes all the parts of our lungs, improves the digestive system, circulatory system and removes problems of the respiratory system, cleans the blood, removes tension, depression, insomnia and heart problems.

The Seven Social Sins

1. Politics without Principles
2. Pleasure without Conscience
3. Wealth without Work
4. Knowledge without Character
5. Commerce without Morality
6. Science without Humanity
7. Worship without Sacrifice

—Mahatma Gandhi

70

Bhastrika (Bellow Breathing)

Bhastrika means the 'bellow instrument' of an iron smith in which air is pumped in and out quickly. Sit in a comfortable posture, inhale and exhale deeply up to the navel region quickly. While doing so, one could mentally recite *Soham*, i.e., I am That (Soul) (I am immortal Soul). While breathing in, mentally recite '*So*' and while breathing out recite '*Ham*'. Do it 10 times.

Take one to two normal breaths. Quickly inhale and exhale up to the chest region, following the *Soham* pattern 10 times. Now breathe normally two to three times.

Now breathe in up to the throat level. Inhalation and exhalation should be very quick. There should be no movement in the body. The feeling of the breath should be only in the nostrils and the throat. Repeat this process of quick breathing 20 times.

Some Yoga Gurus do the *Bhastrika* in the following manner: After two to three normal breaths, keep your fists near your shoulders with elbows touching the sides. Now inhale forcefully and raise your arms up opening the fists. Exhale forcefully and bring your elbows down touching your sides and close your fists. This should be repeated 10 times with the mental recitation of *Soham*.

Bhastrika is useful for liver, kidney, indigestion and stomach-related problems. *Bhstrika* is a tiring exercise. It should be followed by *Ujayyi/Shîtali/Shîtkari Pranayama*. Persons with weak lungs or high blood pressure should avoid it or do it gently. Ladies should avoid this exercise as it puts pressure on pregnancy-related region and chest.

71

Ujayyî Pranayama (Throat-Massaging *Pranayama*)

Sit in a comfortable posture. Close your eyes. Breathe deeply through both the nostrils. Inhalation and exhalation should be felt in the throat. There would be some rustling sound of the breath through the throat and the air going inside should be massaging the throat. There should be no retention of the breath either during or after inhalation or exhalation.

This exercise is good for vocal cords, generating smoothness in voice. It is particularly good for singers. This exercise increases glow of the face and is helpful in insomnia, low blood pressure, mental depression and heart problems. This exercise can be done for 4 to 5 minutes. During the exercise, name of God could be recited by those who believe in Him.

72

Shîtali/Shîtkari Pranayama (Cooling Exercise)

Sit in a comfortable posture. Take out the tongue from the lips and twist it like the beak of a bird and breathe in through the mouth deeply, creating a hissing sound. Retain the breath for a few seconds and breathe out through the nostrils. It may be noted that in *Shîtali Pranayama*, inhalation is through the mouth and exhalation through the nostrils.

There is another similar exercise which is known as *Shîtkari Pranayama* (Cooling Exercise). *Shîtali* and *Shîtkari* both mean cooling. Sitting in a comfortable posture, twist the tongue in your mouth and touch the palatel. Alternatively, the tongue could be pressed against the teeth. Breathe in deeply through the mouth creating the hissing sound. Retain the breath for a few seconds and breathe out from the nostrils.

These exercises should not be done by persons suffering from low blood pressure or pneumonia. In winter, these exercises may be done for a minute or so, in summer, for three to four minutes.

Both the exercises quench thirst and relieve hunger. These are also helpful in heart disease, high blood pressure and insomnia. These exercises add lustre to the face and prevent oral and dental diseases.

73
Kapãl Bhãti (Head-Glow *Pranayama*)

Kapãl means Skull and *Bhãti* means glow, i.e., that which provides glow to the head. It is a *Hatha Yoga Kriya* which is done after *Jal-Neti* (Nasal wash), but as it is *Pranayama*-centric, we have included it in the Breathing Exercise section. Sit steadily and comfortably and place your hands on the knees. Have three normal breaths. And, thereafter, mentally reciting AUM, inhale from both the nostrils slowly and exhale forcefully, quickly and completely. The stomach should contract during exhalation. Exhalaltion should not take more than a second. In this exercise, Retention (*Kumbhak*) is not done. Doing this exercise for three to five minutes is adequate.

Kapãl Bhãti is slightly different from *Bhastrika*. In *Bhastrika*, inhalation and exhalation both are done forcefully. In *Kapãl Bhãti*, force is applied in exhalation, while inhalation automatically follows without any effort. *Bhastrika* is slightly tiring; *Kapãl Bhãti* is comparatively a gentle exercise. Those who feel tired in doing *Bhastrika* or are advised not to do it, should do *Kapãl Bhãti*.

In *Kapãl Bhãti*, all the organs in the head are exercised. Nerves of the brain, eyes, ears and nose are all toned up. This exercise prevents and cures tuberculosis, insomnia and neurological problems. It also adds glow to the face and sharpens memory.

74

Bhrãmari (Bumble Bee) *Pranayama*

Bhramari means a bumble bee. A bumble bee hums around a lotus flower and creates a melodious sound. *Bhramari Pranayama* means creating a humming sound during exhalation.

Sit in a comfortable posture. Close your eyes. Plug your ears with the thumbs so that no outside sound disturbs you. Place the index fingers slightly above the eyebrows and place the other three fingers on the eyes so that the outside light does not affect the eyes. Take a deep breath and without Retention (*Kumbhak*), inhale slowly. Mentally recite *Aum* or any other name of God. Without opening your mouth, emit sound like that of a bumble bee during exhalation. The sound should be like the sound of a church or temple bell, a bit loud in the beginning and receding gradually. Time of exhalation should be double that of inhalation. Rhythm of the *Pranayama* should follow the rhythm of the bumble bee-like sound. 10-12 such breathings are adequate.

Enjoy the sound during *Bhramari Pranayama*. Some flashes of different colours – green, yellow, blue – may appear, enjoy their sight. During *Pranayama*, have the feeling that God's grace is engulfing you. This *Pranayama* is helpful to people hard of hearing, or suffering from high blood pressure, depression, insomnia. *Bhramari Pranayama* is very relaxing and should be done at the end of all Pranayamas. Thereafter, Meditation should be done.

75
Synchronised Breathing – *Pranic* Healing (*Tãrtamay Pranayama*)

Sage Manu has said in the Manusmriti (6.71):

DAHYANTE DHMÃYAMÃNÃNÃM DHÃTUNÃM HI YATHÃ MALÃH

TATHEN-INDRYÃÑAM DAHYANTE DOŠÃH PRAÑASYA NIGRHÃT (136)

i.e., just as the dross of the metals is burnt up by heating the same, similarly, the dross and the toxins of the organs of the body are burnt up by *Pranayama*.

Furthermore, the potency of *Pranayama* is further enhanced by synchronised or rhythmic breathing. What is synchronised breathing? This is a process when the breathing is synchronised with the heartbeat or the pulse-beat. By this process, the breath rate of a Yoga aspirant comes down to nearly 6 breaths per minute as against the normal 15 breaths per minute.

It is scientifically established that the animals that breathe fast die young and the animals that breathe slowly live long. The following table is quite illustrative:

Animal	Breath Rate per Minute	Life-Span (Years)
Tortoise	4	300
Bowhead whale	4-6	200
Elephant	12	100
Man	15	80
Horse	18	50
Dog	24	13

That is why, Rig Veda (1.66-1) says: AYUR NAH PRAÑO NITYO NA SUNÛH (137), i.e., the *Prana* is our life. Meaning thereby, short or deep breaths determines our life span.

Given below is the method for synchronised or rhythmic breathing. Sit steadily in a comfortable posture. Head, neck, chest and spine should be in a straight line. Place hands on the knees and close the eyes, think of Omnipresent God or the vast sky. Have three to four normal deep breaths and relax. Now feel the heartbeat or the pulse-beat. Pulse-beat can be felt by putting fingers on the wrist. And the heartbeat can be felt by putting hand on the heart or palm on the left ear.

For rhythmic or synchronised breathing, please align your one inhalation with six beats of heart or pulse; hold breath for three heart/pulse-beats; exhale for six heart-pulse-beats and retain again for three beats. After a few days, inhalation/exhalation could be increased to eight heart/pulse-beats and retention of breath should be four heart/pulse-beats. Retention should always be half the number of heart/pulse-beats of inhalation/exhalation. To begin with, this exercise should be of three rounds of inhalation, retention, exhalation, retention and could be increased to 7 times gradually. During inhalation/exhalation, mentally recite AUM or Aum Namay Shivaye. Thereafter breathe normally. The exercise should be done morning and evening.

Dr. Deepak Chopra, renowned spiritualist and physician, states, "This synchronising of respiratory and heart rates boosts oxygen in the blood, while improving circulation in the brain."

Synchronised or rhythmic breathing is panacea in all diseases. This exercise removes all respiratory, circulatory, neurological problems and psychosomatic illnesses. It improves memory and intellect and increases life span of the aspirant.

Thus Spake Scholars on India

"O India! Will you not help us?
Be patient with us, India!
Remember, we are your children.
You are old and learned and wise before we existed.
Our path is steep and thorny. Help us Mother India!
We, your real Vedic children, are turning our gaze to our motherland,
Together, we become the great regenerating
and moralising force of the world."

—Lord Flinch

We owe a lot to Indians, who taught us how to count, without which no worthwhile scientific discovery could have been made.

—Albert Einstein

I had been seeing the world in black and white, and when brought face to face with India, experienced everything re-rendered in brilliant technicolor.

—Keith Bellows
(Vice President, National Geographical Society)

Step IV
Meditation

76

Important Observations regarding Meditation

- Meditation is a spiritual process. It is basically a communication with God. It can become really effective, if one has made progress in moral discipline and attained control over mind through *Pranayama*. One should sit for meditation with a composed mind, fixing one's attention on God seated in the Self. St. Augustine's words on this subject are pertinent: "If there is to be effective prayer, the clamour of the senses must cease and urges of the body must stop. It is only then that we can commune in peace with God."
- Please go through the subsection Meditation under Section I – Introduction to Yoga, to recapitulate what exactly Meditation is and what can be achieved by Meditation.
- Directing mind's undivided attention to a particular object or idea is Meditation. In this state, thoughts related to the same subject should appear in the mind and extraneous thoughts should be shut off.
- The subject matter of Meditation could be spiritual or secular. Thinking about God, Soul and Nature or fixing attention on a particular Mantra, Hymn or Ayat is spiritual Meditation. Thinking about material objects and worldly problems is secular Meditation.
- Meditation is both a spiritual and psychological process. With the stilling of mind, spiritual progress as well as peace of mind can be obtained. Researches in psychology have shown that when the mind is still, alpha and theta waves are generated in the mind. In this state, mind's faculties are enlarged including

ability of alpha healing through mental suggestions, auto suggestions.

- Spiritual and positive attitude towards life are essential for progress in Meditation.
- Meditation should be done in early morning or at sunrise or sunset.
- Meditation should be done in a clean, calm and solitary place.
- Before Meditation, Meditation related *Pranayama* should be done.
- Meditation should be done in a comfortable posture; difficult postures are not appropriate for meditation. The sick and old may do meditation in *Shava Asana* (Dead Body Posture).
- Food-related suggestions in Step II and Step III are applicable for Meditation as well.
- Drinking and smoking should be avoided. There is some misconception that smoking and drinking relieve one of tension. In fact, while smoking or drinking, one diverts one's attention from the worries and enjoys the drink or the smoke. It is the act of diversion from the worries, and not the drink or the smoking itself which provides the relief. Meditation is a process of diverting one's mind from the unwanted things and channelising thinking on the desired subject.

77

Trãtaka : Open-Eyed Concentration

The first stage of Meditation is *Dhãrana*, which means retention or concentration. Herein attention is focused on an object or a subject. If attention deviates from the object or the subject, it is refocussed and the object or subject is retained in the mind again. Thereafter, Contemplation (*Dhyana*), the second stage starts.

Trataka is basically a *Hatha Yoga Kriya*. In it, the attention is focussed on an outer object with open eyes. In Patanjali Yoga, there is no provision for focussing attention with open eyes. Attention is always focussed on any object or subject with closed eyes. However, as the beginners may find it easy to focus attention on an outer object with open eyes, we have included Trataka which is helpful for *Dhãrana*. *Trataka* can be done in three ways:

a. Make a round figure on the wall in front of your eyes, exactly parallel. Sit in a comfortable posture. And look at it intently without flickering the eyelids. Even after flickering the eyelids, continue to look at it. Believers may concentrate their attention on AUM or the Cross or the Crescent. When you feel tired by looking at it with open eyes, close the eyes and look at the figure mentally. If it disappears, open the eyes, look at it again for a moment, close the eyes and mentally look at it, retaining it in the mind as long as possible. Repeat this process 3-4 times and, thereafter, only mentally retain the figure and mentally recite AUM or any other name of God. Doing this exercise for about 3 minutes is adequate.

b. Parallel to your eyes, place a candle or a Deepak on some table. The head, the neck, the chest and the spine should be straight. Look at the flame constantly with open eyes. When you feel tired, close the eyes and look at the flame mentally. When it disappears, open the eyes, look at the flame again for a moment and close the eyes. You may simultaneously mentally recite AUM or any other name of God. Repeat this process 3-4 times. About 3 minutes of this exercise is adequate.

c. Sit in a comfortable posture with head, neck and chest in a straight line. Focus your attention with open eyes at the point between the eyebrows. This place is known as *Agya Chakra*. When you feel tired, close the eyes and focus attention on the *Agya chakra* mentally. When the attention deviates, open the eyes and look at the mid-point between the eyebrows for a moment and close the eyes again. Focus attention on the *Agya Chakra* mentally as long as you can. Repeat this process 3-4 times. This exercise is more tiring than the other two. Therefore, 2 minutes of this exercise is adequate. Doing this exercise for an extended period may be harmful.

Trataka is helpful for developing *Dhãrana* or concentration. Those who do not intend to do this exercise with open eyes may do it with closed eyes as per Lesson IV/4. During any of the above *Trataka*, some light of any colour, yellow, blue, green – may appear in the forehead. You may enjoy that light which is indicative of progress in *Dhãrana*.

78

Meditation by Concentration on the Breath

Mind's activities can be stilled just by concentrating on the movement of one's breath. It is not a breathing exercise but making breath as a prop in meditation. This method has been preached by Lord Buddha and this meditation method is known as *Vipãsanã*. *Vipasana* is a Pãli word for Sanskrit word *Vipashyanã*, i.e., act of seeing attentively.

Sit in a comfortable posture. Close your eyes gently. Concentrate on the tip of your nose and be aware of the breath coming in and coming out. No retention of the breath is required. What is required is only to be aware that you are breathing. When you are breathing in, imagine that the energy of the universe and good thoughts and good traits are entering your body and mind. While breathing out, visualise that all the toxins, diseases and infirmities of the body and bad thoughts, bad habits of the mind are going out of your body and mind. Feel calmness and happiness in the mind.

If any thought appears in the mind, just be aware but do not be carried away with it. While breathing in and while breathing out, imagine and say mentally to yourself that I am happy, I am calm, I am in the control of my mind. In so doing, your mind will be stilled and you will enjoy peace of mind and happiness.

79
Meditation by Concentration on Your Forehead (*Ãgya Chakra*)

Sit in a comfortable posture. Gently close your 'eyes and have three deep breaths. Concentrate on your forehead between your eyebrows. This place is known as *Agya Chakra*. Write in golden letters Aum, Allah or God on your forehead. It will disappear, write again. It will again disappear, write again. After some time, some light or flame may appear in the forehead, follow that. That light may change colours – at times, yellow, green, purple or blue colour, do not mind the colour; just enjoy the light and try to retain it as long as you can. Mentally recite the name of God and think of His attributes that He is kind and merciful, omniscient, omnipotent and omnipresent. He is my Saviour. He is enveloping me. I am in His lap. He is protecting me and bestowing grace and bliss on me. No other thoughts should be allowed to creep in. You will enjoy peace and happiness.

80
Meditation by Concentration on Navel *Chakra*

Yoga *Darshãna* (III.29) says: NÃBHI CHAKRE KÃYA VYÛH JNÃNAM (138), i.e., by Meditation on the Navel-disc, one gets knowledge of the body-organization/mechanism.

Sit in a comfortable posture. Close your eyes. Concentrate on your navel region. Mentally observe how the digestive system is functioning properly. Observe how the heartbeats are going on in the regulated manner. Think of the lungs, how the breathing is going on properly. Think of the mind and observe how the thoughts are arising in the mind. But who is responsible for the functioning of this body? We find sometimes that all the parts of the body are intact but there is no movement in any part. The body is called dead. What is that element which has gone out of the body? Is it that which in various scriptures is called *Atman*, Soul, Spirit or 'Ruh'? Surely, I am That – *Soham*. That is why, Descartes arrived at the conclusion 'Cogito Ergo Sum', i.e., I think, therefore, I am.

But I cannot change the functioning of my body. The whole body organism was in place before I was born. How does a child get nourishment in the womb of the mother? Biologists tell us it is through the umbilical cord that is attached to the Navel. But how did my mother sew this umbilical cord (which is cut after birth) when her hands were not in her womb? How has my mother developed my eyes, ears, nose and imbued in them the facilities of sight, hearing and smell? If one's mother was the creator of one's body, no child would have born blind, deaf or crippled. Who has devised this whole mechanism with so much precision? To that supernatural power, commonly known as God, who has devised all this, I bow my head in reverence and admiration. Aum. Aum. Aum.

81
Meditation by Recitation of a *Mantra* or Hymn or *Ayat*

Mind can be stilled and deep-peace felt by recitation of a *Mantra* or Hymn or *Ayat*. Meditating on *Aum* is called *Udgîtha Dhyãn*. While meditating on Aum, one must ponder over its meaning, i.e., Protector. Ãdi Purãna says: NA NÃMA SADRISHAM DHYÃNAM (139), i.e., there is meditation technique which equals meditation on the name of God, i.e., AUM. The Holy Bible: psalm 8.1 also says – "O Lord, Our Lord. How glorious is Thy name in all the earth!" NASA has confirmed that the rays of the Sun emit the sound resembling Aum.

Sitting in a comfortable posture, close your eyes and recite in audible voice *Aum* or *Gayatri Mantra* or *Maha Mritunjaya Mantra*, Allah or any name of God or any *Mantra*, Hymn or *Ayat* in praise of God, thinking at the same time about its meaning, After 5 to 7 loud recitals, the same could be recited mentally. The attributes of God that He is kind, merciful, omniscient, omnipotent and omnipresent should be pondered over along with mental recital.

Listening to the sound of *AUM* or any *Mantra* or Hymn or Ayat recorded on a cassette, at night before sleep will bring in peace of mind and sleep free from unpleasant dreams.

82
Meditation by Concentration on Objects of Nature

Sit in a comfortable posture. Close your eyes. Keep the image of a white lotus flower in the forehead. Think of its beauty and its fragrance. Think how geometrically its petals are arranged and how each petal is artistically designed. It is grown in the mud of a pond. Where from this fragrance and its white, blue or pink colour have come? Think of a rose flower and of a marigold flower. Their colours are different. Their designs are different and their smells are different. All have come out of earth. Where from this difference is colour, design and fragrance has come? All vegetables, fruits are different in taste, different in nutrients, different in smell and appearance. Where from this variety has appeared? It is understandable that fruits and vegetables are grown in the fields and orchards by farmers but who has grown the huge pine trees on the peaks of high mountains where no person has ever treaded?

Surely, there must be some power which is responsible for the functioning of this Nature. I bow my head to that power in reverence and admiration. *Aum. Aum. Aum.*

83
Meditation by Concentration on Sound (*Anãhat Nãda*)

Mind can be stilled by concentrating on any sound. This may be the ripples of a stream, chirping of the birds, whistling of the wind or the rhythmic sound generated by one's own body. Shankaracharya calls it *Anãhat Nãda* and advised SARVA CHINTÃN PARITYAJYA ANÃHATAM SAMÃCHARET (140), i.e., leaving aside all worries, one should meditate upon the *Anãhat Nãda*, i.e., incessant sound.

This world is the creation of God. Poets and saints have found that this Universe is pulsating with some divine music which has been described as Music of the Spheres. Lao Tzu has observed, "The subtle melody of the universal life is eternal and constant, yet only those who are in consonance with it can perceive it." In the Bible, it is said, "In the beginning was the word and the word was with God and the word was God." The scientists also believe that the Universe which was created with a Big Bang still carries the sound of that bang. It is said that Neil Armstrong, the first man on the moon, heard a musical note on the Moon.

Will Durant has said, "We are not sensitive to the overtones of the Reality that hums around us." NASA has now confirmed that the rays of the Sun emit sound resembling the sound of *AUM*.

Sit in a comfortable posture near a stream. Close your eyes and attentively listen to the sound that the running water is creating. Soon you will find that there is rhythm in that sound because the position of stones in the stream is fixed and flow of water is steady. Recite the name of God, *AUM* synchronising with the rhythm and you will enjoy peace. Saint Vinoba Bhave has observed that if a troubled Soul sits near a stream, he gets relieved. Where from the soothing power has come in the murmuring of the stream? God's embalming nature is reflected in it.

Sit in a jungle or in a garden where there is no movement of people. In the solitude, forget your worries and concentrate on the sound being created by the blowing wind. Soon you will find that there is rhythm in the sound. The whistling of the wind would appear musical. Mentally recite the name of God '*AUM*' and synchronise that name with the sound. It will appear as if the wind were singing in praise of God. There is an Irish proverb praying:

"May brooks and trees and singing hills join in the chorus too
And every gentle wind that blows send happiness to you."

Sit in a comfortable posture. Plug your ears by inserting cotton. Close your eyes and don't allow other thoughts to come into your mind. Soon you will listen that in your body, a rhythmic sound is ringing. With that rhythm, synchronise the recital of the name of God, contemplating on its meaning. You will experience peace of mind and happiness.

Thus Spake Sinto-Dinju on God

"The heavens are still; no sound
Where then shall God be found
Search not in distant skies;
In man's own heart He lies."

(Transalated by H.D. Gibbs)
(The Religions of Ancient China)

84
Meditation on Eight *Chakrãs*

In the Atharva Veda, it is stated that in the human body, there are 8 *Chakrãs* and 9 doors. These eight *Chakrãs* are situated in the spinal cord and the head. These are *Mûlãdhãr Chakra* at the anus, *Svãdhišthãn* in the pubic zone, *Manipur* at the navel, *Anãhat* near the heart, *Vishudha* in the throat, *Ãgyã* in the forehead between the eyebrows. *Mãnas Chakra* in the lower brain in the head, Sahasrãr in the head-top, at the joint of the skull.

An invisible *Nadi* (nerve) called *Sushmñã* passes through the spine touching these *Chakrãs*. By meditating on these *Chakrãs*, the *Kundalini* (Dormant Energy) is awakened and vast psychological powers are released.

Sit in a comfortable posture. Close your eyes gently. Withdraw your mind from all worries and thoughts and think of God or the vast sky. Breathing normally, focus your attention or consciousness on any one of the *Chakrãs* where you can easily retain consciousness without wavering. If that is difficult, focus attention on all *Chakrãs* one after the other linking them with a golden line of light. First focus attention on *Mûlãdhãr* onwards up to *Sahasrãr* and then from *Sahasrãr* to *Mûlãdhãr* making a circle of bright light emitting from all the *Chakrãs* like pearls in a necklace. While focussing attention on each, mentally recite the name of God.

While focussing consciousness on *Mûlãdhãr*, visualise that your whole body is being sanctified; while focussing on *Svadhisthan*, visualise that all the baser instincts are being got rid of; while focussing on *Manipur*, visualise that the whole body is being energised; while focussing on *Anahat*, visualise that all the emotions are being controlled; while focussing on *Vishudha Chakrã*, visualise that you are getting rid of ego; while focussing on *Agya Chakrã*, visualise that knowledge is being expanded; while focussing on *Manas Chakrã*, visualise that intuitive power is dawning upon you and while focussing on *Sahasrar*, visualise that you are being engulfed with peace and bliss.

Attention on the *Chakrãs* can also be focussed reciting the following *Mantra*: Aum BHÛH, Aum BHUVAH, Aum SVAH, Aum MAHAH, Aum JANAH, Aum TAPAH, Aum SATYAM. While mentally reciting Aum BHUH, focus attention on *Sahasrar* and *Manas Chakrã* and pray to God for protecting your *Prana*; while reciting Aum BHUVAH, focus attention on *Agya Chakrã* (between the eyebrows), pray for removal of miseries; while reciting Aum SVAH, focus on the *Vishudha Chakrã* (throat) and pray for well-being and prosperity; while reciting Aum MAHAH, focus attention on *Anahat Chakrã* (pit of the diaphragm) and pray for large-heartedness; while reciting Aum JANAH, focus on the *Manipur Chakrã* (Navel) and pray for generating energy in the body; while reciting Aum TAPAH, focus attention on *Svadhisthan* and *Mûlãdhãr* (pubic region in anus) and pray for austerity in life and while reciting Aum SATYAM, focus on all the eight *Chakrãs* aligned in a bright string of light and pray to God to reveal His true nature to you and engulf you in that bright light.

Pregnant women should not concentrate their consciousness on the first three Chakras, viz., *Mûlãdhãr*, at the anus, the *Svadhisthan* in the pubic zone and *Manipur* at the navel as these are the areas which are active in pregnancy and may hamper the growth of the embryo.

85
Meditation on Any Object of Liking

The practice of Yoga is a personal experience for each individual. In meditation, one experiences peace and bliss in his own way. It is difficult to describe such a situation. The sages and saints who have experienced this bliss have not given any details except to state that this is indescribable. Prophet Mohammed has aptly stated:

"There are as many ways to God as Souls,
As many as breaths of Adam's Sons."

Various saints and sages and practitioners of Yoga have indicated ways and means of self-realisation or enlightenment. A few of these have been described in the Yoga *Darshana* of Patanjali.

In this book, we have described some of the methods of practising yoga which have been taught by some teachers and advanced practitioners of Yoga. After describing some of the most prevalent methods of practising Yoga, Sage Patanjali stated YATHÃ ABHIMAT DYÃNÃT VÃ (141), i.e., or by meditating on any object of liking, stillness of the mind is achieved.

The discipline of Yoga is meant for the whole human race and not for any particular race or religion. Individuals professing different faiths can meditate according to their beliefs. They can meditate on Aum or the Cross or the Crescent or God as one conceives Him. All the religions believe that God is one but He is known by different names in different languages and different religions as water is known by different words in different languages. All religions believe God to be kind and merciful, omniscient, omnipotent and omnipresent. Thinking of these attributes of God, one can meditate on any name of God.

Our Christian brethren can meditate by focusing attention on the Cross between the eyebrows. Sit in a comfortable position; close your eyes; have three deep breaths. Visualise Jesus Christ nailed to the Cross. Think of the sacrifice he made for the good of mankind. Think of his preachings like Truth, Love, Compassion, Brotherhood of Mankind and Service of Humanity. And resolve to practice these in your personal life.

Meditate on the hymns related to His grace, kindness and benevolence and pray that He may show you the right path that leads to His eternal home eg

As the hart panteth after the water brooks,
so panteth my soul after Thee, O God!
Preserve me, O God! for in Thee do I put my trust.
Hear, O Lord!, my cry, give ear unto my prayer,
that goeth not out of feigned lips.
Hold up my goings in Thy *Paths,*
that my footsteps slip not.
Show me Thy *Ways,* O Lord! teach me Thy *Paths;*
and lead me in Thy Truth.
Thou art the God of my salvation.
Open Thou mine eyes that I may behold
wondrous things out of Thy Law.
Quicken Thou me according to Thy word.
Remove from me the way of lying.

When your heart genuinely reflects your complete devotion to God, He will listen and shower His grace.

Our Muslim brethren can meditate by concentrating on the Crescent. It is not worship or obeisance to the Crescent but just looking at it mentally as does a devout Muslim look physically at the rising moon on the eve of Îd. Sit in a comfortable posture; close your eyes; have three deep breaths and visualise the Crescent. Think of the greatness, benevolence and mercy of God that He has bestowed on mankind. Mentally recite some Ãyats in praise of God. While concentrating on the crescent in your forehead, think of the vast firmament, the vast Universe, how the Sun the Moon and the Stars are moving in designated path and working for the benefit of Humanity; how they are following His command and they serve as His flags which reflect His power, wisdom (Hikmat) and craftsmanship (Kãrigari). And pray :

Lord of Compassion! All praise unto Thee!
Creator and Protector of the worlds!
Lord God! Beneficent and Merciful!
Master Supreme of the great Judgement Day!
Thee do we serve and Thee beseech for help;
Show us the Path on which Thy blessings rest;
The *Straight Path;* not of those who go astray,
On whom descend Thy wrath and punishment

Also think of God's command :
"I am in your Souls! Why See ye not ?
In every Breath of Yours am I, but ye
Are blind without true eye, and see me not"
Also pray to God :
I have heard and followed your command
I beseech your grace! Afterall we are all to reach you.
Lead us to the right path so that our heart and mind
become pure and we reach you and reside in your lap.

(Quran Sarif's Ãyats 1.4-7, 2.285, 16.12, 22.18, 24.35, 25.61, 31.27, 45.31, 49.7, 55.5, 58.7, 64.1, 87.33, can be meditated upon.)

Even those who do not believe in God can meditate on a snow-covered peak, on the vast expanse of the ocean, on the dancing daffodils in a field or any other object of their liking. Once the mind is concentrated on that particular object, the disturbing thoughts will disappear from the mind and peace will descend.

86
Therapeutic Meditation

In all religions, we find instances where spiritual personalities have healed the sick. While some doubt about the validity of this claim, there is in this phenomenon a spiritual/psychological factor at work. Modern medical scientists are coming around the view that all diseases are related to the mind and can be treated through the mind. When the mind calms down, the severity of the illness is also reduced. Dr. Samuel Johnson had stated, "With an unquiet mind, neither exercise nor diet nor physique can be of any use." In the Yoga *Darshana*, it has been stated that stilling of mind removes illnesses. The modern scientists also believe that in deep sleep or in a state of meditation, alpha and theta mental waves are produced which are helpful in removing illnesses. World-renowned Spiritualist and Physician Dr. Deepak Chopra opines, "Theta Wave: 4-8 Hz, represents the transition from wakefulness to sleep and relates to the subconscious. Increased theta activity is noticed in Yogis who have been practising Meditation for long. Alpha Wave: 8-12 Hz, is associated with relaxation and calm-wakefulness and bridges the conscious and the subconscious states. Normal prayer shows an increase in the alpha activity." These waves can be generated by oneself or by someone who has acquired psychic powers. This is known as alpha healing.

Auto suggestion is yet another method to heal oneself. Seneca has said, "To wish to be well is part of being well." Jess Stearn is also of the view: "The key to your good health and success in life lies in your own subconscious mind, in the type of meditative thinking that produces the slow alpha wave cycles in your brain and enables you to channel your mind and body into positive, creative, healing patterns". – The Power of Alpha Thinking.

Sit in a comfortable posture or lie in *Shava Asana* (Dead Body Posture). Keep your eyes closed and have three deep breaths. Repose faith in God and have unflinchable confidence in yourself. Shower mental waves on the affected part of your body and pray to God to heal it. Make auto suggestion that this particular part of my body is getting well. Mentally also visualise that this part of the body is getting healed as does a modern surgeon heal with his laser beam without actually performing any surgery.

Through this method of concentrating mental awareness on a diseased organ, even a friend or an acquaintance at a distance can be treated by sending mental waves to the affected person. You would have heard the Reiki Healing. It works on this principle. The propounder of Reiki has expressed indebtendess to the Yoga discipline.

Those interested in knowing more on this subject may read the following books:

(a) The Power of Alpha Thinking – Jess Stearn
(b) The Power of Your Subconscious Mind – Dr. Joseph Murphy
(c) Reversing Heart Disease – Dr. Dean Ornish
(d) Pranic Healing – Choa Kok Sui
(e) Psychic Discoveries Behind the Iron Curtain – Sheila Ostrander and Lynn Schroeder

87
Self-Confidence–Related Meditation

(*Manobal Vardhak Dhyana*)

It is a well-known fact that armies with high morale win battles; if their morale is down, the best of weapons cannot help winning the battle. Dr. Joseph Murphy, author of 'The Power of Your Subconscious Mind', states, "A magnetised piece of iron will lift above 12 times its own weight but if you demagnetise this same piece of iron, it will not lift even a feather.... You can become a magnetised person when you discover and put to use the master secret of the ages... This secret is the marvellous, miracle working power found in your own subconscious mind."

Now let us examine, where from does Mind get Self-Confidence? Its source is Soul. Wherefrom does Soul get confidence? It is God. Yajur Veda (25.13) says: YA ĀTMADĀ BALADĀ YASYA VISHVA UPĀSATE (142), i.e., He whom the world worships is the source of physical and moral strength. But whom does God provide this strength? Those who have abiding faith in Him and follow His Laws of Rita and Satya – Moral and Cosmic laws. The Gita (9.22) says: TEŠĀM NITYA-ABHIYUKTĀNĀM YOGAKŠEMAM VAHĀMYAM (143), i.e., those who constantly think of Me, I take care of their safety and prosperity. The Gita also assures: NA HI KALYĀÑ-KRIT KASHCHID DURGATIM TĀT GACHHATI (144), i.e., he who works for the well-being of others does not be get sufferings.

In the Holy Bible (Psalms 16.1, 18.21), there is a prayer:

"Preserve me, O God, for in Thee do I put my trust.

For I have kept the ways of the Lord
and have not wickedly departed from my God."

Armed with the strength of your character and the assurances of the Scriptures, sit in a steady and comfortable posture and have three cycles of rhythmic breathing as advised in Lesson IV/2. Thereafter, mentally recite to yourself

AHAM INDRO NA PARÃ JIGYA IDHANAM
NA MRITVE VA TASTHE KADÃ CHANA (145)

— Rig Veda 10.48.5

(I am Indra, the invincible.
None can conquer my wealth and valour.
Death can never defeat me.)

And give the autosuggestion to yourself:

YATHÃ SURYASHCHA CHANDRASHCHA
NA BIBHÎTO NA RIŠYATAH
EVÃ ME PRÃÑA MA BIBHE (146)

— Atharva Veda 2.15.3

(As the Sun and the Moon
Neither fear nor suffer
So dost thou, my spirit,
Fear not.)

Have firm belief in what Gothe said, "The moment one definitely commits oneself, providence moves too."

Also pray to God: VISHVÃNI DEVA SAVITUR DURITÃNI PARÃ SUVA YAD BHADRAM TANA Ã SUVA (126), i.e., what is evil and harmful, take away from me and what is good and helpful, bring unto me. Also think of Milton's words in Pradadise Lost:

"What in me is dark illumine,
What is low, raise and support."

While going out of the house, have three rhythmic breaths and pray:

MADHU-MANME NIKRAMAÑAM
MADHU-MANME PRÃYAÑAM (147)

— Atharva Veda 1.34.1

(O God! May my going out be sweet,
May my coming back be sweet.)

And mentally create a circle of golden light around yourself with full conviction that it won't be breached and you will remain protected by the grace of God! Aum! Amen! Amin!

Why to Pray?

Prayer opens the spiritual sight of man,
For prayer is desire and desire develops into will.
The magnetic emanations proceeding from the body
at every effort –whether Moral or Physical – produce self
magnetisation and ecstasy.

—H.P. Blavatsky
(Isis Unveiled I, 434)

Prayer is the silent yearning of the soul for affinity
with the Supreme One.

—Plotinus

The object of prayer is not to please God, who does not want our prayers or praise, but to purify ourselves. The process of Self-Purification consists in a conscious realisation of His presence within us. There is no strength greater than that which such realisation gives. Presence of God has to be felt in every walk of life.

—Mahatma Gandhi

88
Contemplative Prayer Healing

(Prayer is Good Medicine)

Yoga *Darshana* (1.29) says: TATAH PRATYAK CHETNÃ – ADHIGAMO APY – ANTARÃY – ÃBHÃVASHCHA (148), i.e., as a result of *Ishvara Pranidhan* (Total Devotion to God), one attains awakening of new consciousness and absence of hindrances like disease, stupor. This scriptural evidence confirms that Prayer/Devotion to God has a healing effect.

It is not our claim that the broken bones can be joined by prayer. Nor do we claim that the host of diseases can be cured by prayer alone without using medicines. The emphasis here is to quote Karen S. Judd, "Taking a spiritual approach to life promotes healing." God has provided a self-healing mechanism in the body. Greek philosopher Hippocrates has opined, "Natural forces within us are the healers of diseases. Healing is a matter of time, but it is also a matter of opportunity." Prayer only hastens the process of healing.

Dr. Larry Dossey, the author of 'Prayer is Good Medicine', cites studies proving that concentrated thought could inhibit the growth of fungi, yeasts and bacteria. Another study says wounded mice prayed for healing faster.

World-renowned spiritualist and physician Dr. Deepak Chopra has analysed this phenomenon thus: "When we have a thought or feeling, our brain produces neuropeptides or nerve proteins that send chemical messages to other cells in the body. Prayer helps produce serotonine, a neuropeptide, that positively influences mood and behaviour. The healing process starts here."

Dr. Deepak Chopra further states rituals such as prayer positively impact the immune and cardiovascular systems. For instance, Prof. Luciano Barnardi of the University of Padwa, Italy, says, "Reciting of Yoga *Mantras* and Ave Maria slows the respiratory rate to 6 breaths a minute, which coincides with the rhythmic oscillation of nervous impulses controlling the heart rate. This synchronicity of respiratory and heart rates boosts oxygen in the blood while improving circulation to the brain."

Dr. Deepak Chopra poses a pertinent question: 'Can a petition made to God cure diseases?' and answers "Science has been searching for a conclusive answer. But the idea that the mind can effect the body has been prevalent for a long time in eastern and western traditions. There are studies showing that those who pray contemplatively, or meditate, can positively influence their health. For instance, the very act of prayer makes a person sit quiet, release tension and let go of stress. This in itself has a positive physiological effect."

Dr. Deepak Chopra further explains what happens in the brain when you pray, "Parietal lobe helps us distinguish ourselves from the world. This part of the brain is associated with orientation and gives a person a distinct sense of individuality – the sense of 'I'. During prayer, this area becomes quiet as a result the distinction between self and the world disappears. Frontal lobe is associated with individual will. Prayer modulates brainstem manoamine nuerotramsmitters like dopamine and norepinephrine, helping a person let go of ego. Prayer and meditation also cause frontal and temporal lobe circuits, which mark time and self-awareness to snap. Your immune system is continually eavesdropping on your internal dialogue."

Prof. Alexis Carrel has also opined, "Prayer is the most powerful form of energy one can generate. The influence of prayer on the human mind and body is as demonstrable as that of the secreting glands. Prayer is a force as real as terrestrial gravity. It supplies us with a flow of sustaining power in our daily lives."

To sum up, during one's own illness or of one's dear ones, one must pray for early recovery and it will yield amazing results.

Nobel Laureate Alexis Carrel on Prayer

"A tranquillity of bearing, a facial and bodily repose,
are observed in those whose inner lives are enriched by prayer.
Within the depth of consciousness a flame kindles.
And man sees himself.
He develops a sense of moral obligation, intellectual humility.
Thus begins a journey of the soul towards the realm of grace."

89

Total Devotion to God – *Ishvara Pranidhana* (Does God Listen to One's Prayers?)

Ishvara Pranidhana is not a meditation process. It is a state of total devotion and surrender to God and while walking, eating or doing anything, always keeping one's mind fixed on God. It is a state of mind like that of a child lost in a fair, where no amount of sweets and toys now please him; he is incessantly crying to meet his mother. To such persons, God does listen. St. Augustine's words on this subject are pertinent: "If there is to be effective prayer, the clamour of the senses must cease and urges of the body must stop. It is only then that we can commune in peace with God."

Given below are two real-life incidents which went viral on social media in April 2017.

First relates to Heart Surgeon in Baroda (Gujarat). He said that a couple brought to him a girl of six years whose heart was completely clogged. He told them that there were 30% chances of her survival in an operation, otherwise the child has only three more months to live. The couple requested the Doctor to go ahead with the operation. Before the operation the Doctor told the child, "Do not be afraid, you will be alright." The child replied, "I am not afraid. God resides in the heart. When you open my heart, please see God and tell me how he looks."

During the operation, it was found that nothing can be done because there was not a single drop of blood in her heart. The Doctor stated, "In frustration, I asked my team to stitch the heart back. At that time, the last words of the child came to my mind. And with bloodstained folded hands, I prayed: O God! My whole experience is not able to save this child. If you are there in her heart, you do something."

"This was my first tearful prayer. During this time, my junior nudged me. I did not believe in miracles. But I was dumb-founded to see that blood supply had started in the heart. This happened for the first time in my 60 years' career."

The Doctor further said, "Operation was successful, but my life got changed. I told the child God cannot be seen, it can only be experienced. After that incident, we started praying regularly in the operation theatre. I urge that parents should inculcate the *Sanskara* (habit) of praying among their children."

The second incident relates to the renowned Heart Specialist, Dr. Trehan of Medantha of Gurugram. He caught a flight to attend some conference. After some time, the pilot announced that due to heavy gale and rough weather, the aircraft will be landing at the nearest airport. On emergency landing, Dr. Trehan complained to the pilot, that his presence at the conference was very necessary. Somebody recognised him and told him that he could catch some taxi and will be able to reach his destination within three hours. Thanking the person, he took a taxi.

Due to heavy rain and storm, the driver lost the way. They reached a lonely place and found shelter in a house where an old woman was reciting Sukhmani Sahib of Guru Granth Sahib. Dr. Trehan sought the permission to use her phone. The old woman replied, "Beta, there is no phone or electricity here. Drink some water and I will prepare something to eat."

While drinking water, Dr. Trehan noticed that during her recital of Sukhmani Sahib, she was occasionally shaking the child sleeping near her. Dr. Trehan said, "Amma, I am deeply impressed with your devotion to God. I wish you also pray for me. I am sure, God will listen to your prayer."

The old woman replied, "Beta, there is nothing of that sort. I always pray for Sarbat Ka Bhala, e.g., may all be well. God has fulfilled all my prayers. I am only now praying for one more favour." "What is that, the Doctor asked. She replied, "This child who is lying near me is totally dependent on me. His father and mother both are dead. In this old age, how can I look after him? He is suffering from a severe disease. Doctors say they cannot treat him. They say there is only one famous Doctor who can treat him. What is his name? Yes, Dr. Trehan. I, old woman, how can I reach him? I am only praying to God to resolve my difficulty."

Hearing this, tears started flowing from the eyes of Dr. Trehan. He spoke in a choking voice, "Amma, your prayer generated lightening and storm in the sky and made the aircraft to make a forced landing. Your prayer made me forget my way and attracted me to your house. O God! I can't believe it! How can Vaheguru (God), to listen to the prayer of His devotee, can help in this way!"

Inscrutable are the ways of God. He not only listens, He also speaks. Sage Aurobindo said, "Eternity speaks, but no one listens."

Prayer or Miracle?

It has been said that "The usual influence of Christian belief" (and indeed of all blind belief, in any religion) "has been to override the idea of invariable causation in nature; even after the belief in recurrent miracles is disavowed, the doctrine and practice of prayer remain to represent the old concept" : (**J.M. Robertson**, A short history of Christianity Pg 242); the old concept, viz, that God can intervene, to change the ordinary course of causation, in answer to prayer. (The Essential Unity of All Religions, Pg 576: Dr. Bhagwan Das)

90
Experiences (*Anubhûti*) During Meditation

In *Samadhi* or deep state of meditation, when the mind has fully withdrawn from the worldly objects and is concentrated on the inward realities, the practitioner experiences extreme peace and happiness. Albert Einstein has aptly commented, "The most beautiful and most profound emotion we can experience is the sensation of the mystical." In this state, the practitioner attains certain divine powers and sees divine visions. In the hour of meditation, the practitioner sees lights of various colours – red, purple, yellow, green, blue – floating in his forehead. Sometimes, even in waking state, he sees these lights roaming around in his vicinity. At times, in the state of meditation, his body becomes light and he even feels that the spirit has left his body and after roaming around for some time, it re-enters the body. In fact, in this state, his astral body goes to the different places and gets information. In the hour of mediation, sometimes the practitioner sees some enlightened persons or has vision of world-renowned Messengers of God like Buddha or Christ blessing him and guiding him for progress in the spiritual path. Sometimes, the practitioner smells some fragrance without the presence of any flower or incense stick in his vicinity. Sometimes, he listens to some divine music coming from the space or can have knowledge about any incident past, present or future.

These are some of the divine powers which the practitioners acquire during their progress on the path of Yoga. The practitioners are advised not to exhibit such powers or talk about these as this will hinder their progress on the spiritual path. Such occurrences take place only to assure the practitioner that he is on the right track and will at some distant future get enlightenment, the goal of Yoga.

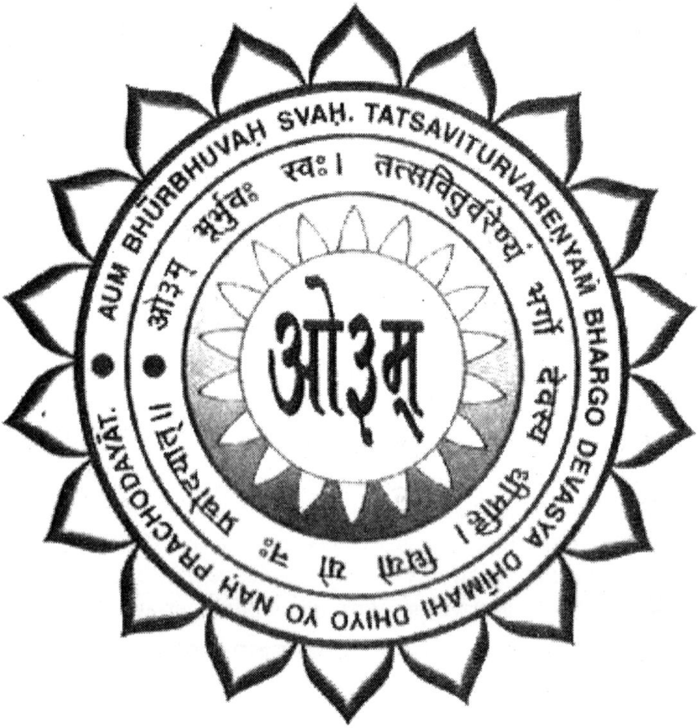
AUM BHŪRBHUVAḤ SVAḤ. TATSAVITURVAREṆYAṀ BHARGO DEVASYA DHĪMAHI DHIYO YO NAḤ PRACHODAYĀT.
ओ३म् भूर्भुवः स्वः। तत्सवितुर्वरेण्यं भर्गो देवस्य धीमहि। धियो यो नः प्रचोदयात्॥
ओ३म्

गायत्री मन्त्र

ओ३म् (रक्षक ईश्वर) भूः (प्राणदाता) भुवः (दुःखहर्ता) स्वः (ऐश्वर्य का दाता) तत् (उस) सवितुः (जगत् रचयिता) वरेण्यं (वरण करने के योग्य) भर्गः (तेजस्वरूप) देवस्य (देवता का) धीमहि (ध्यान करते हैं)। धियो (बुद्धि को) यो (जो-उपरोक्त) नः (हमारी) प्रचोदयात् (पवित्र करे)

तूने हमें उत्पन्न किया, पालन कर रहा है तू ।
तुझ से ही पाते प्राण हम, दुःखियों के कष्ट हरता है तू ॥
तेरा महान् तेज है, छाया हुआ सभी स्थान ।
सृष्टि की वस्तु-वस्तु में, तू हो रहा है विद्यमान ॥
तेरा ही धरते ध्यान हम, मांगते तेरी दया ।
ईश्वर ! हमारी बुद्धि को, श्रेष्ठ मार्ग पर चला ॥

Annexture
(अनुबन्ध)

मूल संस्कृत उद्धरण

1. तत्सवितुर्वरेण्यं भर्गो देवस्य धीमहि।
   धियो यो नः प्रचोदयात्॥ —ऋग्वेद 3.62.10

2. अग्ने नय सुपथा रायेऽअस्मान् विश्वानि देव वयुनानि विद्वान्।
   युयोध्यस्मज्जुहुराणमेनो भूयिष्ठां ते नमऽउक्तिं विधेम॥
   —यजुर्वेद 40.16

3. यस्येमे हिमवन्तो महित्वा यस्य समुद्रं रसया सहाहुः।
   यस्येमाः प्रदिशो यस्य बाहू कस्मै देवाय हविषा विधेम॥
   —ऋग्वेद 10.121.4

4. युजे वां ब्रह्म पूर्व्यं नमोभिर्वि श्लोकऽएतु पथ्येव सूरेः।
   शृण्वन्तु विश्वेऽअमृतस्य पुत्राऽआ ये धामानि दिव्यानि तस्थुः॥
   —यजुर्वेद 11.5

5. असतो मा सद्गमय।
   तमसो मा ज्योतिर्गमय।
   मृत्योर्मा अमृतं गमय। —बृहदारण्यक उपनिषद्

6. सहस्राह्ण्यं वियतावस्य पक्षौ हरेर्हंसस्य पततः स्वर्गम्।
   स देवान्त्सर्वांनुरस्युपदद्य सपश्यन् याति भुवनानि विश्वा॥
   —अथर्ववेद, 10.8.18

7. योगश्चित्तवृत्तिनिरोधः। —योगदर्शन I.2

8. मन एव मनुष्याणां कारणं बन्धमोक्षयोः। —ब्रह्मबिन्दु उपनिषद्–2

9. शरीरमद्य खलु धर्मसाधनम्। –कालिदास

10. संयोगो योग इत्युक्तो जीवात्मपरमात्मनोरिति। –याज्ञवल्क्य

11. आत्मानं विधि –उपनिषद्

12. ध्यायतो विषयान्पुंसः सङ्गस्तेषूपजायते। –गीता 2.62

13. वसुधैव कुटुम्बकम्। –पंचतन्त्र

14. विर्तकबाधने प्रतिपक्षभावनम्। –योगदर्शन 2.33

15. स्थिरसुखमासनम्। –योगदर्शन 2.46

16. द्वाविमौ वातौ वात आ सिन्धोरा परावतः।
दक्षं ते अन्य आ वातु परान्यो वातु यद्रपः॥

–ऋग्वेद 10.137.2

17. चले वाते चलं चित्तं निश्चले निश्चलो भवेत्। –प्रकीर्ण

18. प्राणाद् वायुरजायत। –ऐतरेय आरण्यक

19. प्राणो वै बलं तत् प्राणे प्रतिष्ठितम्। बृहदारण्यक उपनिषद् 5.14.4

20. त्रिवृद्वै प्राणाः। –तैतरेय आरण्यक 5.4.11

21. बाह्याभ्यान्तरविषयाक्षेपी चतुर्थः। –योगदर्शन 2.51

22. तज्जयात्प्रज्ञाऽऽलोकः। –योगदर्शन 3.5

23. प्रकृत्यापूरात्। –योगदर्शन 4.2

24. दिवि सूर्यसहस्रस्य भवेद् युगपदुत्थिता। –गीता 11.12

25. नीहारधूमार्कानिलानलानां खद्योतविद्युत्स्फटिकशशीनाम्।
एतानि रूपाणि पुरःसराणि ब्रह्मण्यभिव्यक्तिकराणि योगे॥

–श्वेताश्वतर उपनिषद् 2.11

26. अनेकजन्मसंसिद्धस्ततो याति परां गतिम्। –गीता 6.45

27. द्वा सुपर्णा सयुजा सखाया समानं वृक्षं परि षस्वजाते।

तयोरन्यः पिप्पलं स्वाद्वत्त्यनश्ननन्यो अभि चाकशीति।

—ऋग्वेद 1.164.20,

28. महो अर्णः सरस्वती प्रचेतयति केतुना।
धियो विश्वा वि राजति।। —ऋग्वेद 1.3.12

29. कारणाभवात् कार्याभावः। —वैशेषिकदर्शन 1.2.1

30. ब्रह्मणस्पतिरेता सं कर्मारइवाधमत्।
देवानां पूर्व्ये युगेऽसतः सदजायत।। —ऋग्वेद 10.72.2

31. रचनानुपपत्तेश्च नानुमानम्। प्रवृत्तेश्च। —वेदान्तदर्शन 2.2.1-2

32. यो विद्यात् सूत्रं विततं यस्मिन्नोताः प्रजा इमाः।
सूत्रं सूत्रस्य यो विद्यात् स विद्याद् ब्राह्मणं महत्।।

—अथर्ववेद 10.8.37

33. मयि सर्वमिदं प्रोतं सूत्रे मणिगणा इव। —गीता 7.7

34. ऋतं च सत्यं चाभीद्धात्तपसोऽध्यजायत। —ऋग्वेद 10.190.1

35. अश्रद्धामनृतेऽदधाच्छ्रद्धाᳬं सत्ये प्रजापतिः। —यजुर्वेद 19.77

36. नेश्वराधिष्ठितेफलनिष्पत्तिःकर्मणातत्सिद्धेः।

—साख्यदर्शन 5.2

37. पूर्वेषामपि गुरुः कालेनानवच्छेदात्। —योगदर्शन 1.25

38. शास्त्रयोनित्वात्। —वेदान्तदर्शन 1.3

39. यदाऽऽत्मतत्त्वेन तु ब्रह्मतत्त्वं दीपोपमेनेह युक्तः प्रपश्येत।
अजं ध्रुवं सर्वतत्त्वैर्विशुद्धं ज्ञात्वा देवं मुच्यते सर्वपाशैः।।

—श्वेताश्वतर उपनिषद् 2.15

40. स्वप्ननिद्राज्ञानालम्बनं वा। —योगदर्शन 1.38

41. समाधिसुषुप्तिमोक्षेषु ब्रह्मरूपता। —साख्यदर्शन 5.116

42. एकं सद्विप्राः बहुधा वदन्ति। —ऋग्वेद 1.164.46

43. अवति रक्षति इति ओ३म्।

44. एक एव नमस्यः। –ऋग्वेद

45. सर्वे अस्मिन् देवा एकवृत्तो भवन्ति। –अथर्ववेद 13.4.21

46. क्लेशकर्मविपाकाशैरपरामृष्टः
पुरुषविशेष ईश्वरः। –योगदर्शन 1.24

47. स पर्यगाच्छुक्रमकायमव्रणमस्नाविरꣳशुद्धमपापविद्धम्।
कविर्मनीषी परिभूः स्वयम्भूर्
यथातथ्यतोऽर्थान् व्यदधाच्छाश्वतीभ्यः समाभ्यः।।
–यजुर्वेद 40.8

48. अपाणिपादो जवनो ग्रहीता पश्यत्यचक्षुः स शृणोत्यकर्णः।
स वेत्ति वेद्यं न च तस्यास्ति वेत्ता तमाहुरग्र्यं पुरुषं महान्तम्।।
–श्वेताश्वतर उप. 3.2

49. सहस्त्रशीर्षा पुरुषः सहस्त्राक्षः सहस्त्रपात्।
स भूमिꣳसर्वत स्पृत्वात्यतिष्ठद्दशाङ्गुलम्।। –यजुर्वेद 31.1

50. न तस्य प्रतिमाऽअस्ति यस्य नाम महद्यशः। –यजुर्वेद 32.3

51. न ज्येष्ठासः न कनिष्ठासः एते। –शतपथ ब्राह्मण

52. तत् त्वमसि। –छान्दोग्य उपनिषद् 6.9.4

53. त्वं स्त्री त्वं पुमानसि। –श्वेताश्वतर उपनिषद् 4.3

54. तासामनादित्वं चाशिषो नित्यत्वात्। योगदर्शन 4.10

55. ईश्वरः सर्वभूतानां हृद्देशेऽर्जुन तिष्ठति।। –गीता 18.61

56. आत्मनि ब्रह्म। –शांखायन आरण्यक

57. अन्ति सन्तं न जहात्यन्ति सन्तं न पश्यति। –अथर्ववेद 10.8.32

58. तमेव विदित्वाति मृत्युमेति नान्यः पन्था विद्यतेऽयनाय।
–यजुर्वेद 31.18

59. जन्मादिव्यवस्थातःपुरुषबहुत्वम्। –सांख्यदर्शन 1.149

60. ममैवांशो जीवलोके जीवभूतः सनातनः। –गीता 15.7

61. निवसिष्यसि मयि एव –गीता

62. अंश इवांशो न हि निरवयवस्य
मुख्योऽशः सम्भवति। –आदिशंकराचार्य

63. जीवो ब्रह्मेति नेतरः। –आदिशंकराचार्य

64. सत्त्वरजस्तमसां साम्यावस्था प्रकृतिः। –साख्यदर्शन 1.61

65. सर्वं त्रैराशिकं पाती। –प्रकीर्ण

66. नाशः कारणलयः। –साख्यदर्शन 1.121

67. अदितिर्द्यौरदितिरन्तरिक्षमदितिर्माता स पिता स पुत्रः।
विश्वे देवा अदितिः पञ्च जना अदितिर्जातमदितिर्जनित्वम्॥
–ऋग्वेद 1.89.10

68. तत् सन्निधानादधिष्ठातृत्वं मणिवत्। –साख्यदर्शन 1.96

69. मयाध्यक्षेण प्रकृतिः सूयते सचराचरम्।
हेतुनाऽनेन कौन्तेय जगद्विपरिवर्तते॥ –गीता 9.10

70. अनुपभोगेऽपिपुमर्थं सृष्टिः। –साख्यदर्शन 6.40

71. भोगापवर्गार्थं दृश्यम्। –योगदर्शन 2.16

72. ब्रह्मसत्यं जगद्मिथ्या। –आदिशंकराचार्य

73. न सद्रूपानासद्रूपा मायानैवोभयात्मिका।
सदसद्भ्यां निर्वाच्या मिथ्याभूता सनातनी॥

74. नाभाव उपलब्धेः। –वेदान्तदर्शन 2.2.28

75. मायां तु प्रकृतिं विद्यान्मायाविनं तु महेश्वरम्।
–श्वेताश्वतर उप. 4.10

76. एतज्ज्ञेयं नित्यमेवात्मसंस्थं नातः परं वेदितव्यं हि किंचित्।
भोक्ता भोग्यं प्रेरितारं च मत्वा सर्वं प्रोक्तं त्रिविधं ब्रह्ममेतत्॥
–श्वेताश्वतर उप. 1.12

77. बृहत्वात् ब्रह्म।

78. स नो बन्धुर्जनिता स विधाता। –यजुर्वेद 32.10

79. क्रतुमयः पुरुषः। –वेद

80. मनुष्याः कस्मात् मत्वा कर्माणि सीव्यन्ति। –निरुक्त 3.8.2

81. अवश्मेव हि भोक्तव्यं कृतंकर्म शुभाशुभम्। –उपनिषद्

82. कर्मण्येवाधिकारस्ते मा फलेषु कदाचन।
मा कर्मफलहेतुर्भूर्भा ते सङ्गोऽस्त्वकर्मणि॥ –गीता 2.47

83. न हि कश्चित्क्षणमपि जातु तिष्ठत्यकर्मकृत्। –गीता 3.5

84. कर्मण्यकर्म यः पश्येदकर्मणि च कर्म यः।
स बुदिमान्मनुष्येषु स युक्तः कृत्स्नकर्मकृत्॥ –गीता 4.18

85. संस्कारो हि गुणान्तराधानमुच्यते। –ऋषि चरक

86. केवलं ग्रहनक्षत्रं न करोति शुभाशुभम्।
सर्वमात्मकृतं कर्म लोकवादो ग्रहा इति॥ –महाभारत अनु.पर्व 145

87. जानामि धर्मं न च मे प्रवृत्तिः जानाम्य धर्मं न च मे निवृत्तिः।
केनापि देवेन हृदिस्थितेन यथा नियुक्तोऽस्मि तथा करोमि॥
–महाभारत

88. स इह स्थानेषु प्रत्याजायते यथाकर्म यथाविद्यम्।
–शांखायन आरण्यक 3.2

89. देवत्वं सात्त्विका यान्ति मनुष्यत्वं च राजसाः।
तिर्यक्त्वं तामसा नित्यमित्येषा त्रिविधा गतिः॥ –मनुस्मृति 12.40

90. शरीरजैः कर्मदोषैर्याति स्थावरतां नरः।
वाचिकैः पक्षिमृगतां मानसैरन्त्यजातिताम्॥ –मनुस्मृति 12.9

91. नाभुक्तं क्षीयते कर्म जन्मकोटिशतैरपि। –उपनिषद्

92. तिष्ठेत् कर्मफलं यावद् व्रजेत कर्मक्षये पुनः। –उपनिषद्

93. पुनर्मनः पुनरायुर्मऽआगन्पुनः प्राणः
पुनरात्मा मऽआगन्पुनश्चक्षुः पुनः श्रोत्रं मऽआगन्।
विश्वानरोऽअदब्धस्तनूपाऽअग्निर्नः पातु दुरितादवद्यात्॥
–यजुर्वेद 4.15

94. मृतश्चाहं पुनर्जातो जातश्चाहं पुनर्मृतः।
नानायोनिसहस्राणि मयोषितानि यानि वै॥ –निरुक्त 13.19

95. जातस्य हि ध्रुवो मृत्युर्ध्रुवं जन्म मृतस्य च। –गीता 2.27

96. ये मृताः सहसा मर्त्याः जायन्ते सहसा पुनः।
तेषां पौराणिको भावः कञ्चित् कालं हि तिष्ठति॥
–महाभारत अनुशासन पर्व 145

97. प्रेत्याहाराभ्यासकृतात् स्तन्यभिलाषात्। –न्यायदर्शन 3.1.22

98. पूर्वाभ्यस्तस्मृत्यनुबन्धाज् जातस्य हर्षभयशोकसम्प्रतिपत्तेः।
–न्यायदर्शन 3.1.19

99. यद्गत्वा न निर्वतन्ते तद्धाम परमं मम। –गीता 15.6

100. पुरुषार्थ चतुष्ठय।

101. अथ त्रिविधदुःखात्यन्तनिवृत्तिरत्यन्तपुरुषार्थः। –साख्यदर्शन 1.1

102. द्रष्टृदृश्ययोः संयोगो हेयहेतुः। –योगदर्शन 2.17

103. बाधनालक्षणं दुःखम्।
तदत्यन्तविमोक्षोऽपवर्गः॥ –न्यायदर्शन 1.1.21-22

105. ईशा वास्यमिदꣳसर्वं यत्किञ्च जगत्यां जगत्।
तेन त्यक्तेन भुञ्जीथा मा गृधः कस्य स्विद्धनम्॥
–यजुर्वेद (40.1) ईशोपनिषद्-1

106. कुर्वन्नेवेह कर्माणि जिजीविषेच्छतꣳ समाः।
एवं त्वयि नान्यथेतोऽस्ति न कर्म लिप्यते नरे॥
–यजुर्वेद (40.2) ईशोपनिषद्-2

106. यज्ञार्थात्कर्मणोऽन्यत्र लोकोऽयं कर्मबन्धनः।
तदर्थं कर्म कौन्तेय मुक्तसङ्गः समाचर॥ –गीता 3.9

107. ऋषिः स यो मनुर्हितः। –ऋग्वेद 10.26.5

108. अनावृत्तिः शब्दात्। –वेदान्ह दर्शन 4.4.22

109. न मुक्तस्य पुनर्बन्धयोगोऽप्यनावृत्तिश्रुतेः। –साख्यदर्शन 6.17

110. न च पुर्नावर्तन्ते। –छान्दोग्य उप 8.15.1

111. यावत् ब्रह्मलोकस्थिति तावत्तत्रैव
तिष्ठति प्राक्ततो नावर्तत इत्यर्थः। –आदिशंकराचार्य

112. ते ब्रह्मलोके ह परान्तकाले परामृतात्
परिमुच्यन्ति सर्वे। –मुण्डक उपनिषद् 3.2.6

113. इदानीमिवसर्वत्रनात्यन्तोच्छेदः। –सांख्य 1.159

114. ते तं भुक्त्वा स्वर्गलोकं विशालं
क्षीणे पुण्ये मर्त्यलोकं विशन्ति। –गीता 9.21

115. मोक्षस्य न हि वासोऽस्ति ग्रामविशेषः। –शिवगीता

116. सति मूले तद्विपाको जात्यायुर्भोगाः। –योगदर्शन 2.13

117. उत्तिष्ठत जाग्रत प्राप्य वरान् निबोधत। –कठोपनिषद्

118. अष्टादशपुराणेषु व्यासस्य वचनं द्वयम्।
परोपकारःपुण्याय पापाय परपीडनम्॥ –प्रकीर्ण

119. यदग्ने स्यामहं त्वं त्वं वा घा स्या अहम्।
स्युष्टे सत्या इहाशिषः॥ –ऋग्वेद 8.44.23

120. यस्तन्न वेद किमृचा करिष्यति। –ऋग्वेद

121. न तस्य रोगो न जरा न मृत्युः।
प्राप्तस्य योगाग्निमयं शरीरम्॥ –श्वेताश्वतर उप. 2.12

122. स्वस्ति पन्थामनु चरेम सूर्याचन्द्रमसाविव।
पुनर्ददताघ्नता जानता सङ्गमेमहि॥ –ऋग्वेद 5.51.15

123. धृतिः क्षमादमोऽस्तेयं शौचामिन्द्रियनिग्रहः।
धीर्विद्यासत्यमक्रोधो दशकं धर्मलक्षणम्॥ –मनुस्मृतिः 6.92

124. आत्मनः प्रतिकूलानि परेषां न समाचरेत्। –महाभारत

125. द्वौ संनिषाद्य यन्मन्त्रयेते राजा तद् वेद वरुणस्तृतीयः।
–अथर्ववेद 4.16.2

126. विश्वानि देव सवितर्दुरितानि परा सुव।
यद्भद्रं तन्नाऽ सुव॥ –यजुर्वेद 30.3

127. योऽस्मान् द्वेष्टि यं वयं द्विष्मस्तं वो जम्भे दध्मः॥
–अथर्ववेद 3.27.1

128. भोजनान्ते विषम वारिः। –प्रकीर्ण

129. सर्वेषामेव रोगाणां निधानं कोष्ठबद्धता। –प्रकीर्ण

130. आ यन्मा वेना अरुहन्नृतस्य
एकमासीनं हर्यतस्य पृष्ठे। –ऋग्वेद 8.100.5

131. सूर्यऽआत्मा जगतस्तस्थुषश्च। –यजुर्वेद 7.42

132. कालं वञ्चनार्थाय कर्म कुवन्ति योगिनः। –प्रकीर्ण

133. शौचात्स्वाङ्गजुगुप्सा परैरसंसर्गः। –योगदर्शन, 2.40

134. अग्ने यन्मे तन्वाऊनं तन्मऽआपृण। –यजुर्वेद 3.17

135. बाह्याभ्यन्तरविषयाक्षेपी चतुर्थः। –योगदर्शन, 2.51

136. दह्यन्ते ध्मायमानानां धातुनां हि यथा मलाः।
तथेन्द्रियाणां दह्यन्ते दोषाः प्राणस्य निग्रहात्। –मनुस्मृति 6.71

137. आयुर्न प्राणो नित्यो न सुनूः। –ऋग्वेद 1.66.1

138. नाभिचक्रे कायव्यूहज्ञानम्। –योगदर्शन, 3.29

139. न नामसदृशं ध्यानम्। –आदि पुराण

140. सर्वचिन्तान् परित्यज्य अनाहतं समाचरेत्। –आदिशंकराचार्य

141. यथाभिमतध्यानाद्वा। –योगदर्शन, 1.39

142. यऽआत्मदा बलदा यस्य विश्वऽउपासते। –यजुर्वेद 25.13

143. तेषां नित्याभियुक्तानां योगक्षेमं वहाम्यहम्। –गीता 9.22

144. न हि कल्याणकृतकश्चिद् दुर्गातिं तात् गच्छति। –गीता 6.40

146. अहमिद्रो न परा जिग्य इद्धनं
न मृत्यवेऽव तस्थे कदा चन। –ऋग्वेद 10.48.5

146. यथा सूर्यश्च चन्द्रश्च न बिभीतो न रिष्यतः।
एवा मे प्राण मा बिभेः॥ –अथर्ववेद 2.15.3

147. मधुमन्मे निक्रमणं मधुमन्मे परायणम्। –अथर्ववेद 1.34.3

148. ततः प्रत्यक्चेतनाधिगमोऽप्यन्तरायाभावश्च। –योगदर्शन, 1.29

149. सुखस्य मूलं धर्मम्।
धर्मस्य मूलमर्थम्।
अर्थस्य मूलं राज्यम्। –चाणक्यनीति

150. माता भूमिः पुत्रोऽहं पृथिव्याः। –अथर्ववेद, 12.1.12

151. अग्नि मीळे पुरोहितं यज्ञस्य देवमृत्विजम्।
होतारं रत्नधातमम्॥ –ऋग्वेद, 1.1.1

About the Author

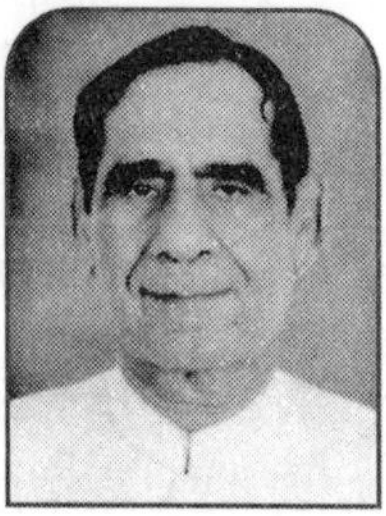

Shri Vidya Sagar Verma is a retired Indian Foreign Service officer (1974 Batch). He served as Ambassador, to Kazakhstan, High Commissioner to Papua New Guinea, Deputy High Commissioner to Australia and Deputy Director General Indian Council for Cultural Relations (ICCR), apart from diplomatic assignments in Afganistan, Egypt, Fiji and Iran.

He studied Sanskrit and Philosophy at graduation level and obtained Masters Degree in English Literature from Panjab University Chandigarh.

His personal library comprises the 4 Vedas, 108 Upnishads, 6 Darshanas, the Gita, the Japaji Saheb, Dhamapad the Holy Bible, Quran Sharif and many books on Indian and Western Philosophy.

When he was High Commissioner in Papua New Guinea, he authored Yoga Darshana : Kavya Vyakhya—a Poetical Commentary on Yoga Sutras of Maharishi Patanjali, released by the Hon. Vice President of India, Shri Krishna Kant in April 2002.

In Kazakhstan, Ambassador Verma conducted Yoga classes in the Embassy, free of charge, for Kazakh nationals and Diplomats. Over 1500 persons were imparted training in Yoga.

His lectures on Yoga were compiled in a bilingual book 'Lessons in Practising Yoga' (English and Russian).

He also got translated the Gita, 1100 Mantras of Rig Veda and abridged Mahabharata in Kazakh language. On his recommendation, Translator Prof. Aubabir Nilibaye, was awarded Padama-Shri by the Hon. President of India in January 2004.

Shri Vidya Sagar Verma has been associated with Samkalp since 2010. He was awarded Guru Samman by Samkalp in July 2015.

Tel: 0120-2395102/9871724733
Email: vidyasagar.verma@gmail.com

About the Book

'Lessons in Practising Yoga' is a comprehensive book on the philosophy of Yoga and how to practise it. Yoga is the workshop of Indian Philosophy and the soul of Indian Culture. For the proper understanding of what Yoga is and what its purpose is, the book covers, in detail, the whole gamut of Indian philosophy comprising the Trinity of God, Soul and Nature and the Triad of Bondage of Karma, Reincarnation of Soul and Liberation. Ashtanga Yoga of Maharishi Patanjali is essentially a spiritual discipline. Accordingly, the book lays due emphasis on Moral Discipline and Meditation. The book contains tips as to how to elevate oneself spiritually and how to meditate, apart from how to do the Yoga-Asanas and Pranayama exercises. The book is replete with relevant quotations of renowned philosophers and scientists as also references from the scriptures of major Religions of the world. The book stresses the universality of Yoga, stating that Yoga is both spiritual and secular. Those who meditate on material subjects attain knowledge of worldly matters as did Newton discover the Law of Gravity. And those who meditate on spiritual matters, advance spiritually as did Swami Dayanand Sarasvati, Swami Vivekananda and Yogi Aurobindo Ghosh.. Rev. Albert Mohler Jr. said "You may be twisting yourself into pretzels or grass-hoppers, but if there is no meditation or direction of consciousness, you are not practising Yoga".The world today is perched on a mountain of nuclear weapons and any misadventure on the part of some egocentric world leaders may annihilate human existence on earth. Yogic prescriptions will calm down their surcharged tempers and will generate feelings of well being of humanity. The words of French philosopher Romain Rolland deserve the attention of the world leaders: "Yoga is the gift of the ancient times, even of unearthly civilisation and if we do not use the knowledge of millennia, we will lose one of the chances for survival".